Letters for my Little Sister

Cecilia Buyswheeler Gunther

and The Fellowship

with Melissa Hassard

Copyright 2014 © Cecilia Buyswheeler Gunther
All rights reserved.

This book or any portion thereof may not be reproduced or used in any manner whatsoever without the express written permission of the author.

Cover and interior design by Sable Books
Cover art by Kathryn Sparks

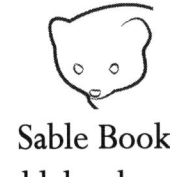

Sable Books
sablebooks.org

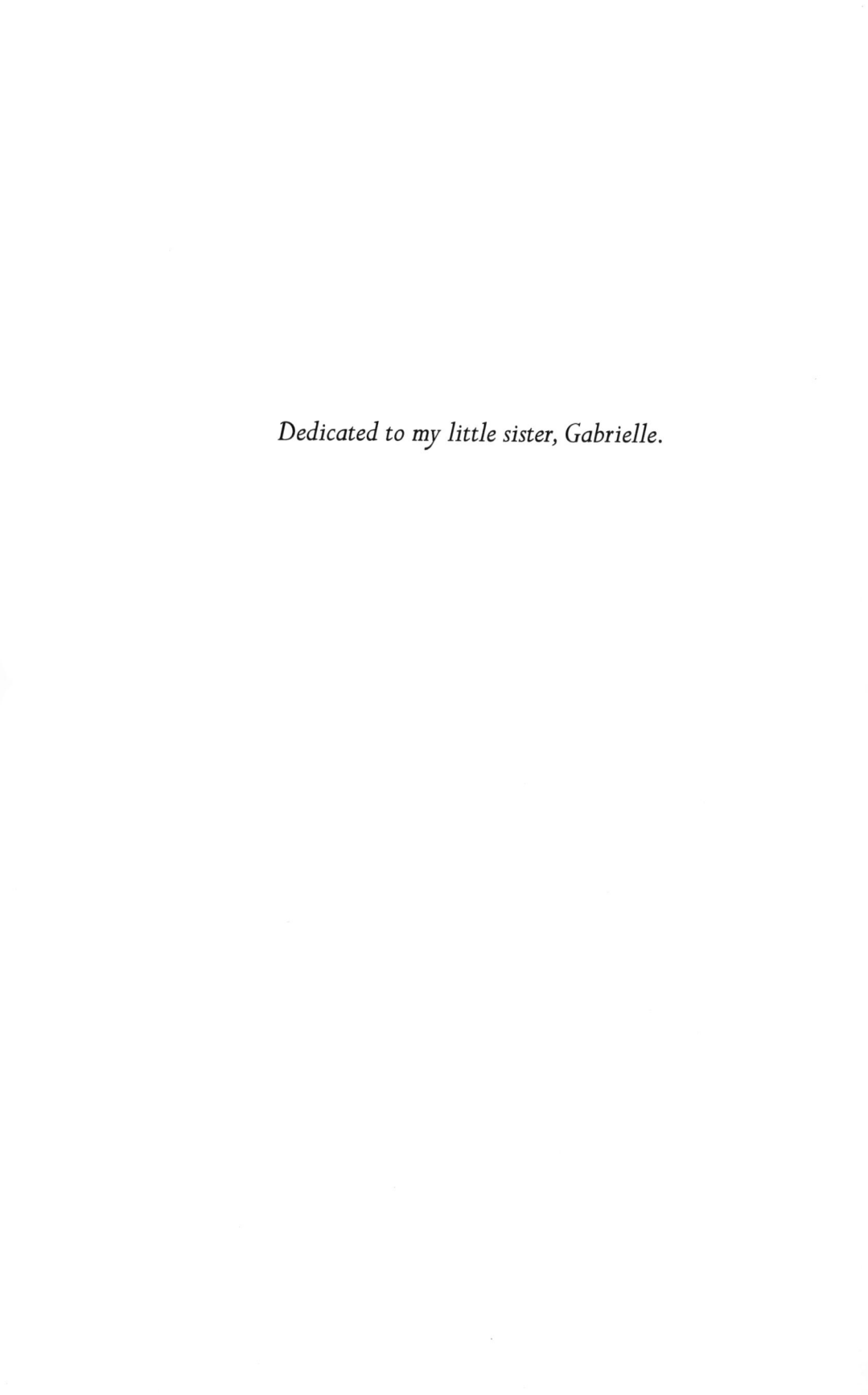

Dedicated to my little sister, Gabrielle.

Foreword

The book you are about to read is a collection of letters written for my little sister. The letters are all about menopause. They are all personal. All anecdotal. All real. There are no lectures, no speeches, no indulgent pompous words. No editors, or spin doctors or page polishers. Just real ordinary people like you and me telling our stories about The Change. Glimpses of real life.

It all began when I sat down to write a letter to my little sister to try to let her know what to expect from menopause. Our mother died long ago without mentioning anything; my grandmother, who died soon after, certainly never discussed these things; and so I had no female familial hook to hang my questions on. Reading about it on Google skips the whole gaggle-of-crones step. As I stared at the page, I realized I had no idea what I would say to my sister to help her through this next period in her life.

So, I asked my friends on my farm blog. This may sound like an unusual place to ask for help about menopause, but on my little farm blog there are a most amazing group of women and men—old farmers, current farmers, city dwellers, nomads, lovers of life and *people*. Off the land, on the land and from all around the world, they are all OF the land. And they are Kind. Kindness is a vastly underrated quality. I call my friends on the blog; 'The Fellowship' of The Farmy. They are "The Fellowship."

I asked The Fellowship if they could tell me how menopause had treated them and what I should know, and with a great Roar of Delight, they sprang into action. The response was instant and intense. The pens and pages flew. It was like a dam breaking. Many, many women wanted to talk. They wanted to share.

I realized that, quite by mistake, we had a book. A real book.

A book! Well I had never had one of those before, and I swiftly concluded that I was now officially out of my depth. I run a small sustainable farm, growing my own food, from big animals to small animals to huge vegetable gardens. I write a little, produce a daily farm blog page, but I am much better at milking my cow, raising chickens on pasture, feeding calves, fattening my vegetarian pigs and gardening. I really needed help.

That is a wonderful thing about life; if you keep your eyes open and your head up you will often see the person that you need or the challenge you should take, right there beside the road along which you are speeding. Often they are holding up a big flashing metaphorical sign in case you do not take the hint. This has happened so often in my life that I have learnt to stop my metaphorical little buggy and say hop right in. This is how I found Melissa Hassard who has co-compiled this book with me.

And so this book was begun.

As I read the written works in this little book, it occurred to me that menopause is a solitary challenge for a woman. Puberty has books and school lessons and magazines, periods even have adverts and smiling girls attached. Everything pink and perky. (Or blue for the squeamish). Once your period arrives you are a woman, overnight and forever more. TADA! Brilliant, isn't it?

But menopause, an equally important time, is possibly a more difficult time because it is often a very rocky journey, sitting all Martha Stewart Beige and slightly nauseous with a headache in the Antique Room with the curtains pulled, kind of ignored. Hidden.

Menopause needs to come into the light. This is the period when we step with womanly power into our third quarter. The third act in our play. One of the richest quarters for a woman, because now her inner artist moves gently in her bourgeoning belly, and she starts to work for herself. But climbing this ladder into this gentler period of female strength is a lonely, and sometimes difficult, path. There are no heralds, there is no applause. No graduation. No flowers. It is slower, crueler, fraught with sagginess, sadness, and goodbyes, but laden with rich promise that we can choose to lift to our drifting breasts and nurture. Or not.

Time and time again, I read that our mothers and grandmothers never talked about menopause; even our grandmothers' mothers and their grandmothers never talked about it. I think we wish there was a wonderful club that spoke openly about these things. In a world of mass media and massive information it is time to change this theme of pretending that menopause means old. Old means old. Menopause is a PAUSE not an ending. We pause. We regroup. We will soon begin again. And in so doing, when we pick up this promise, we shake out all the jewels we have been quietly collecting over the years in our lifetime's pockets and we start to make something with them.

However, in the end, after the last glass of wine or perhaps before the first cup of coffee, menopause, and all its changes, is something a woman must manage within herself. And she can, I can, You can. We can do that. With a glance or a word, we can share our journey, but it seems we seldom do. So we must find ways to allow the youthful, fertile part of our lives to slowly move over and be carefully replaced with our new harder-won, well educated creative lives. The growth and nurturing of ourselves through our homes, our people, our gardens, our art, our sewing, our writing, our travel, our Selves. Now, after menopause has done its worst and for some woman it is a rigorous unrelenting trial, it is finally a Woman's time. This is my challenge to me. To find the time. To get past the rough times. To be that woman.

Some of the most important pages in this book are blank. You will find them after the last letter. These blank pages are waiting for you to write your story in your words, with your voice. Then when you pass this book along to your daughters or nieces or granddaughters or your own little sisters, your story will go along in the book too and together we will build a bridge to help our glorious women out of the brown antique room and into the sun to start kicking some creativity around.

Much love.

Cecilia Buyswheeler Gunther

thekitchensgarden.com

P.S. I have to add a word of caution here. It is very easy for us to read The Letters, draw parallels with our own lives, and flick strange symptoms aside attributing them to menopause. This is not always the case. This is not a medical journal. We will not tell you how to be or how to cope. Every menopausal journey is different. This is a group of women sharing experiences. So always, check with your medical professional if you are at all alarmed. Find a lovely doctor who will listen to you.

celi

Letter from Melissa

Before I started reading these letters, I knew next to nothing about menopause beyond the well-noted hot flashes and attendant moodiness that are the conventional wisdom. But as I began working with the letters and essays included in this manuscript, it struck me that I recognize myself in many of the passages. I have some of the requisite moody days when I feel weepy or emotional. My body's cycles are becoming irregular.

What I love most about this project is that it allows so many women to share their experiences with those who are grateful to hear them. We as women, from a very tender age, learn that our bodies definitely control much of our experience. Being a woman means you hold mysteries inside of you, mysteries even unto yourself. Menstruation, breasts, sex, pregnancy, giving birth, post-partum, and menopause – all of these are mostly unfathomable until we experience them, and we look for answers in books, and in the advice and experiences of family and friends. I am grateful for the wisdom in these pages.

I am 43 years old and it's difficult to separate the changes in my personal life from the changes in my body – but as I read the stories in this book, it seems that is true for many women. One of the messages in this book is – *you are not alone.*

Listen to your body, and follow your heart.

With much love,

Melissa Hassard

Contents

Cecilia (Part One) — 1
One (Laverne Thomas Doyle) — 7
Two (Esther Bradley-Detally) — 8
Three (Marilyn 'Misky' Braendeholm) — 10
Four (Barb Bamber) — 11
Five (Diann Dirks) — 16
Six (Linda Gay Brown) — 21
Seven (Debra Kaufman) — 22
Eight (Faye Blondin) — 24
Nine (Juliet Batten) — 27
Ten (Amanda King) — 30
Eleven (Ella Dee) — 31
Twelve (Beth Ann Chiles) — 34
Thirteen (Maggie O'Connor) — 38
Fourteen (Sandy Wyatt) — 40
Fifteen (Leigh Tyler Olsen) — 41
Sixteen (Ardys Zoellne) — 43
Seventeen (Anonymous) — 46
Eighteen (Karen W. Parker) — 48
Nineteen (Debra Kaufman) — 52
Twenty (Linda Gay Brown) — 53
Twenty-One (Kate Chiconi) — 55
Twenty-Two (Kim) — 58
Twenty-Three (Bela Johnson) — 62
Twenty-Four (Charlotte Moore) — 70
Twenty-Five (Elise K) — 75
Twenty-Six (Grandma Farreline) — 78
Twenty-Seven (Marilyn) — 79
Twenty-Eight (Virginia Bassett) — 81
Twenty-Nine (Melinda S. Roepke) — 83
Thirty (Laura) — 85
Thirty-One (Katy Lamb) — 86
Thirty-Two (Barb) — 87
Thirty-Three (Lyn) — 94
Thirty-Four (Janine Ann) — 96

Thirty-Five (Lori Lynn)	98
Thirty-Six (Nancy Anderson)	101
Thirty-Seven (Grannymar)	104
Thirty-Eight (Sharyn Dimmick)	109
Thirty-Nine (Jean)	110
Forty (Mandy Frielinghaus)	111
Forty-One (Susan)	113
Forty-Two (Debbie Tecca)	115
Forty-Three (Robin Simmons)	118
Forty-Four (Betsy)	121
Forty-Five (Debra Kaufman)	123
Forty-Six (Christine M. Kaess)	129
Forty-Seven (Teri Ridley)	130
Forty-Eight (Debbie)	132
Forty-Nine (Bev DiBell)	134
Fifty (Auntie Eunice)	135
Fifty-One (Misky)	138
Fifty-Two (MarmePurl)	139
Fifty-Three (Janet Knight)	140
Fifty-Four (ViV Blake)	141
Fifty-Five (Marla Eversole)	143
Fifty-Six (Teresa Elliott)	145
Fifty-Seven (Debra Kalka)	146
Fifty-Eight (GA in GA)	147
Fifty-Nine (Mona Baker)	149
Sixty (Debra Kaufman)	152
Sixty-One (Cheerio)	153
Sixty-Two (Eha Carr)	156
Sixty-Three (Joy)	159
Sixty-Four (Alison B)	160
Sixty-Five (Melissa DeCarlo)	162
Sixty-Six (Kathryn Sparks)	164
Sixty-Seven (Sheryl Rider)	168
Sixty-Eight (Beth Kennedy)	174
Cecilia (Part Two)	175
Your Letter	185

In every woman there is a Queen.
Speak to the Queen and the Queen will answer.

Norwegian proverb

Letters for my Little Sister

Cecilia (Part One)

Spring
The Prairies of Illinois
USA

It is morning here. The cool crisp time of day when the air is still owned by the birds. I have milked my cow and fed the pigs, calves and chooks the milk, moved sheep and run dogs, caught runaway chickens (three to go), fed seventy-six chicks (many of whom are destined for the pot), weeded one garden and mowed one lawn, raked the hay driving my little green John Deere tractor (I hate raking the hay, there is a secret to it and no one is sharing). I sowed another round of courgette and cucumbers, started another cheese and now—with my second cup of coffee of the day (my first is at 4:30a.m.) on the windowsill, Tima (the kunekune pig who reminds me of home) asleep on my foot with his two minders, the dogs, optimistically asleep by the doors—finally, it is time to sit in my writing chair by the cool North windows and write you Your Letter.

It is time we had our motherly talk about The Menopause. We are that age now. And it is Spring.

My cows are belly deep in grass. As you are sliding into winter over there in New Zealand, we have leapt into late spring, and it is a wonderful place on the Prairies in the spring. I have lived here seven years now, far from any family, thousands and thousands of miles from my own grown children, and yet, even though the sadness of this never really leaves me, I do love this little farm. I feel a frisson of delight when the plants start to grow again after our killing winters. Where you are, in New Zealand, the land I will always call home, it happens ever so slowly, an organic swell of seasons in and out like sleeping breath. Here in the Americas, like many things on the prairies, the seasons change with a Shout. The plants thrust themselves up from the ground growing at an alarming rate, and fruit massively for a short manic number of weeks. Then it all changes gear, slowly dying, before you know it there is nothing but cold empty fields and stripped gardens. It is the cycle. Our cycle. A bit like our bodies, I suppose. We all live with cycles. Cycles are pretty cool. Except bicycles, I have never been fond of them. The Menopause has cycles within cycles and all of them are quite normal. You will see this when you get to read the letters my friends have written for you. Yes, we have ALL written to you!

Now that we are in our fifties (and someone please explain how that happened), you and I not only need to think about The Menopause but what comes next. Menopause is a gateway through which we will all venture. We can look back a little. There is a lot to be said about actually taking the lid off our muddled minds and objectively peering down into our lives. Poking at them with a long stick. It takes some work to keep a life on the rails. And as we chug along like good little trains, it is so easy to forget—or maybe we choose to forget— that we will not always be deliciously young, with our pale transparent freckly skin and our wild hair and our grandmother's ice blue eyes. So after we have peered back into the well of our past lives, we need to stand up and look forward too. We need to work out how to transition into mature ways. We need to think about these things. More importantly, we need to make sure that the track on which we are chugging is the track we chose to be moving along. Sometimes the lines are switched while we are sleeping. You have to watch out for that.

Looking forward, in relation to our bodies and the demands our bodies make on our minds, it is easier if we can ask elders of our family. However, you, our Middle sister, and I have no mother, or grandmothers, to help us along the way. In fact, these people have been dead for many years now.

So, I have been trying to remember Mum at this period in her life in case we can learn from her dealings with menopause. Though she never grew to be as old as we are now, she did live through her forties, and so I suspect there were symptoms of menopause mixed in there. How far her body got into the cycle of menopause before the cancer interfered, I am not sure. However, I am sure that it had begun. She was a woman. Menopause is a womanly thing. This is why it is so beautiful and so devastating. It has a daunting power.

I wish I had asked Mum why she was so angry during that period. I wonder if she asked herself. If ever there is a scream for help, it is often amplified by anger. There is always an underlying reason. Menopause aside. When you are angry, there is a reason. A teenager's untidy bedroom does not turn a rational person into a screaming heemy-meemy.

Our Mum never talked about menopause, but I think that she just never got around to it; she was open about most things. Well, some things.

When our mother told me about sex, she spelt it aloud S-E-X. She could not say the word. I was perched on the end of her bed. The morning sea breeze blew reflected sun into her big airy bedroom making it glow with that particular promising brightness you only get at the beach. She was in her changing room, getting dressed for something. She was always going somewhere, and she always dressed well: stockings, heels, powder, and lipstick. She was talking to me, but the curtain of her changing room was shut. So I got the whole sex talk from a quiet disembodied voice behind heavy floral fabric. She began the standard talk about vaginas and penises. Sex before marriage will scar you for life, ruin your reputation, sullied goods, etc., you know, the usual stuff, you probably had the same talk.

Then her voice kind of rose and she said, "Bad girls call it a Bad word." Here she paused, a heavy uninterruptible pause, her deeply puritanical Catholic white gloves and pillbox hat persona struggling with the horror of having to think about the bad word. "Well," she finally said, "it rhymes with Suck." Silence. The floral curtain swayed as she moved about amongst her collection of clothes. "You must never use this word." she strained her voice.
"S-E-X?" I asked, spelling it for her.
"No." she replied, her voice pitching from side to side as she shook her head. The sound of hangers clanking against each other, the whoosh of cloth, the slip of her silk

petticoat.

"The one that rhymes with Suck," she said. She carried on talking but by now, she had lost my attention completely. I was casting about in my mind for a word that was bad and rhymed with suck and where could I get me one. The irony was completely lost on me then. The suck thing. I bet she wished she had never started that little thread of intrigue.

However, she said nothing about menopause. And why would she. We girls were being trained to be good wives and mothers who would have lots of babies and keep a good Catholic household. If we wanted to work, we were gently directed to teaching or nursing. The arts and music were encouraged, (they were the gentle arts after all) but the fact that one day we would no longer be fertile and our thoughts would drift elsewhere and god help us all we might even become old women behaving badly, was not in her repertoire.

She forgot to add that after that frantic period of fecundity, our bodies would burn the fields, and all those seeds of the plans we'd been neglecting for years would have a chance to grow. A chubbier version of our prepubescent dream life would be allowed to see the light again. Poor old Mum died without knowing of these things I suppose.

I am off, out to pick my lunch. When I was weeding this morning, I noticed that the beetroot needed thinning. I will selfishly thin all these little seedlings (complete with baby beetroots) into my salad bowl, add some torn up kale, baby spinach, parsley and walnuts. I have some left over potatoes too, I might cut one of those in, add a boiled egg then a small dollop of my favourite mayo. The hand blender one. Eggs, grape seed oil, mustard, garlic, green herbs, pepper and salt. Blend, blend. Chill. Chill. Back soon.

celi

One

When I was growing up, my Mother would always 'dress-up' to go out; high heels, hose, nice dresses (no such thing as pants, Levis or slacks to go 'shopping') nice hair, lipstick and mascara, white gloves, hat, sparkly earrings and necklaces, maybe even a broach on her jacket or coat, just to go to the grocery store.

Gradually, we grew older. Menopause came for my mother. While visiting my parents (they had moved to Hayden, Colorado, by this time)…Momma (always a lady until the day she died) said she had to have a break… she took her cigarettes (yes she also smoked until the day she died) and me, and we sat out on the back step while she puffed vigorously. The sweat was pouring off her face. Then she exhaled slowly and looked at me.

If anyone tells you menopause is easy, she said quietly, wearily…*smack them in the mouth.*

LaVerne Thomas Doyle

Two

My mom was racked by horrible menopause, but Lord knows we didn't speak of bodily functions, so besides her agony of too much sensitivity, shock treatments to get rid of alcoholism and she had endured menopause, a bruised word that hung in closets and hallways of our 12-room house in West Roxbury, Massachusetts. Fast forward to her early death (massive stroke) and her daughter discovering California with its emphasis on youth and hormone replacement therapy.

Reader, I breezed through menopause. That was before warnings of HRT chugged down the pike. Speed back to my being twelve, and flat chested, and lurch through my high school years where I was voted Most Popular, but never, ever, ever wore a sweater to school.

Menopause? I grew after hormone replacement therapy. No sweats, no intense moods — because I was intense and felt everything since I was seven. Later, after heart surgery, blah, blah, all illness which might be discussed by this writer at eighty, I had sweats.

I "grew" is a word we girls in the 50's used. Add that to a period referred to as "my friend," and anything happening "below the waist," and "down there," and you'll catch my drift. I had the gloom of menopause hanging on some epigenetic hook, and alcoholism and depression in a nearby closet. Civilization creaks forward, and because my time was not my mother's time, I had therapy, meds, programs, a plethora of solutions. It isn't perfect, and I feel like an old Studebaker whose doors fall off at a touch, but I am here to tell you, over the edge, getting into older is worth it. Physically and in many other ways, life is hard, but insight and wisdom and landing on a planet – the *Now I Know Who I Am* – is worth it.

Esther Bradley-Detally

Three

Warm Greetings from Menopause

There tucked into early night,
when barking dogs give up their voice,
and streetlights flicker off to dark,

There fleshed into December chill,
when snow hurried thick through the air,
and I was deep in slumber's flock,

There on that snowy December night,
I woke in storms of August heat. Lank
and damp, I breathed in fiercely hot,

I changed my bedclothes, changed
the sheets. All I touched, so sodden through,
and I asked, had I died and gone to hell!

But all was fine, yes, quite well. T'was
just Warm Greetings from Menopause…

Marilyn 'Misky' Braendeholm

Four

Never underestimate yourself, dear.

I had my babies a bit late in life compared to my girlfriends. My daughter arrived when I was thirty-two and my son was born two years and thirteen days later. After so many tumultuous years of baby and toddler juggling with work scheduling nightmares, I asked my husband to have a vasectomy and much to my relief he complied.

Life's challenges didn't let up, my husband would get up, eat the breakfast that I'd made for him and leave us to go to his Big Job downtown. Despite being a quiet introvert with the patience of Job, I found my patience wearing bone-thin and I'd scream at my beautiful babies to get into the car every morning. Not because I was angry, but because I would be late for my own Smaller Job as a classroom teacher. How had I turned into this Monster, surely it must have been the nights of disturbed sleep, demands from work and the daily grind of everyday life? I decided to chalk it up to that. I was exhausted.

One day, my period just stopped, I was forty-three years old, so I thought I'd better get in to see my doctor who was also a family friend. Dr S. gave me a suspicious once-over when I asked for a pregnancy test. I told her that the vasectomy must have failed because I hadn't had my period for three months. I'll admit a secret part of me was hoping I could be pregnant. The test came back negative and I'm sure my doctor thought I must be having an affair if I was so convinced I must be pregnant.

I kept feeling something was amiss; I'd go months without a period and I kept buying pregnancy tests, but every time that little magic wand read negative. Around that time, I watched an Oprah show about menopause with Christine Northrup. I remember sitting up and mentally checking off every symptom they mentioned.

Back I went to the doctor where I was reassured that I was much too young for menopause and that hormone levels can fluctuate any time throughout a monthly cycle. Undeterred, I finally went to a Walk-In Medical Clinic and was sent for more blood tests. They called me back a few days later to go over the results. I'll never forget the young doctor reading through the results, struggling to figure out why my hormone levels were so low. Then, with a shocked voice, he looked at me and said, "You're in menopause."

I knew it then, I think I had known it all along, despite being so young. I thought menopause happened at sixty! But that was the first time I knew I needed to trust myself, to trust my intuition… no matter what anyone else tells you.

My mother had a hysterectomy at a young age, so there wasn't much information for me there, but lots of support! Fortunately, a girlfriend of mine was going through it at exactly the same time. We were so uninformed, but one thing we both concurred was that we were feeling incredibly depressed. This was a very unexpected symptom of menopause. I had always been so upbeat, positive and contented. This was a definite change and red flag for me. After the tension and anger of the early years peri-menopause years, came this deep depression. Both of us vowed we would rather face the risks associated with HRT than feel depressed like that for the rest of our lives. At that point, we were thinking quality of life mattered more. On a side note, I think the connection between hormones and depression needs further investigation. When you hear about postpartum depression resulting from dropping estrogen levels, doesn't it make sense that the same thing could happen at menopause?

I was given the option of taking antidepressants or HRT. I figured at least my body was used to estrogen and progesterone, unlike antidepressants that would be foreign and potentially have side effects. I also chose to undergo prescription, rather than "natural" Hormone Replacement Therapy alternatives and didn't have any difficulty with it. Short, small boned and fair women tend to have issues with bone density and the HRT helped with my osteopoenia.

But there's the whole emotional component to address here as well. I feel as though the estrogen hormone that my body produced until my mid forties was a nurturing hormone. I was focused on how I could best love and care for those around me. I was self-sacrificing and generous. I wonder if our bodies are actually physically designed (for the most part) to be nurturing during childbearing years?

After menopause, it was as though I experienced a rebirth. I often think of the Sleeping Beauty metaphor of being awakened after a long sleep, only it wasn't a prince that woke me up this time! I definitely became less focused on those around me and could finally really see myself, my life and the people in it with so much more clarity. As the estrogen decreased, I felt the need to realign and focus on myself and my own desires, rather than worrying about how I should fit in with the rest of the world. I began wondering how the rest of the world would begin fitting in with me. My own exploration and journey became a new priority, a new focus. It was liberating. It was empowering. It still is.

I drew a line in the sand and began saying, "I'm fifty now, so I don't have to or want to do that anymore." I decided to no longer accept or tolerate anything that wasn't positive or beneficial to my own personal well being. This is when I began teaching myself how to draw boundaries to protect my own best interests. I will admit, I almost "threw the baby out with the bathwater" at one point because I felt such an urgent need to reinvent myself. I was welcoming back and reacquainting myself with the young woman I once was, before I became a wife and mother.

Those years of boundary making have evolved into this new period of recognizing that there are events that happen in life that we can't change and people that we can't control. I'm learning to let go. When faced with a recent difficulty, I realized that none of it occurred as a result of something I had done. In the past I would have wondered what I had done wrong. I now recognize that, in these sorts of situations, sometimes none of it is something I could change or fix. All I could do was focus on how I could respond to the situation. So I chose to step back from the "mess" and reevaluate what was important to me, I discovered those things in my day-to-day life that I could control and that gave me joy. I discovered that true joy for me is very simple: family, friends, learning, creativity and being physically active.

Having gone through this is almost like going through a "gauntlet," it's difficult, it's frustrating, it's scary, you can feel so alone, but it is so worth it. Now I feel strong and know that whatever life throws at me, I can handle it on my own. Fortunately, with family and friends I won't have to go it alone, but if I had to, I know I'd be okay. There's so much to be grateful for in knowing that.

These years have been the most creative and powerful years of my life. Now I ask myself what I want first, then see how it can work with those around me. If I want to try something new, I do it without fear of embarrassment or failure.

I used to be a small puzzle piece that was trying to fit into someone else's big puzzle. Now I'm creating my own puzzle, inventing it as I go along and choosing the shape and size of pieces I want to insert into the beautiful life "puzzle" I am making.

Just this past week, I decided I'd had enough HRT. For no reason at all, it just felt like it was time. I waited for the panic attacks and night sweats to start up again, but there's been absolutely nothing... except when I drink wine – but I'm not giving that up!

It's still early, but I think I'm on the other side now. Time will tell ... or my intuition will!

Barb Bamber

Five

Dear Celi's sister,
I'm sixty-eight now and went through menopause starting an early forty-eight. But I had a homeopath who turned it around and extended things for about eight years. However, my mom died when I was nineteen so I didn't have anyone to talk to me about it. The symptoms startled me at first and I didn't recognize them – feeling flushed and warm suddenly, face flushing. I always had intermittent periods so being irregular didn't surprise me or make me worry. At first, my symptoms were terrible – and I opted for a homeopath, and not an M.D. – who, in my opinion, would have put me at serious risk for cancer by giving me horse urine hormone replacement therapy. I felt like my nerves were on fire. Everything was annoying to me, like bristly hairs of aggravation all over me. It was awful. I wanted out of my skin. The homeopathy worked wonders, and I returned to menses. Later it started again but not severe as before, and a medical doctor gave me mild birth control pills he said were all-natural. They were not, and it took my homeopath to rid me of the side effects again. (I learned my lesson about M.D.'s finally, thankfully.) The fake stuff in those pills bind to the receptors in the body and screw things up royally for a lot more than hormones – they alter communication within the body for many things, none of them good.

Then I was in a place I couldn't get the homeopath's help for sixteen months and I really went through it finally. It was quite difficult for me at the time because I was going through a lot of anxiety because of something I was trying to accomplish, with many barriers in my way. I'd wake up in the middle of the night and just moan from frustration, worry, etc., much of it only amplified by the hormone changes. Eventually that passed.

But here comes the good news. Although the sex drive has slackened off to nothing with me, and sex can be annoying because of dryness and a bit of pain, the body still likes it, just not so often. But the other thing is that I realized for years those hormones and the sex drive really ruled my life. Monthly stuff aside, the desire to be sexy, pretty, attractive, etc. were important to me. It also made me grumpy every month, gave me headaches, put a craving in the body that made me do some really stupid things, especially earlier in my life as a young woman. It was at times pretty overpowering. That left with the monthlies and I was darned glad. At first I missed my womanly processes, but later it was so nice not to worry about wearing white clothing, carrying pads and having to remember to take herbs and such every month.

But as I have matured into a post-menopausal woman (isn't it weird how we classify ourselves by our sex rather than by our intellectual or achievement selves), my life has become so much richer, and happier in so many ways. Okay, so I can't run everywhere like I used to, but that's only because old knee injuries have interfered. I usually have tremendous stamina. The emphasis of my life has shifted greatly. So much of my time and effort these days is about helping people, using my wisdom to be of help to younger people adrift or needing stability and good advice, and now I have the wisdom to offer that help or not, and not be offended if it is rejected. I can grant people to be themselves and just enjoy them and admire them as they are.

I've expanded my curiosity about so many things, have the time to explore and research, write, work on my projects. The list of things I now do is amazing. I let my status as an elder of the tribe work for me. It doesn't take being a Native American to be an elder. You just assume the status and let it go before you. People in the South are very kind to older people and give us help and care unlike the west coast where I used to live. I'm called "Miss Diann" and I love it.

I'm willing to listen to people and hear what they need and what they don't say. It comes with experience. And I'm free to spend hours on the Internet researching things I have become passionate about. This has led to me doing a lot of writing, many smaller books and in progress; a couple of full length works relating to my passions of natural environmental design (Permaculture Design), 1700's medicine and history, and organic gardening. I have time to devote to groups working on things I find important, like my local library, my 1700's Living History Society, my Ladies Homestead Gathering, and several groups and farmers markets, community gardens and sustainability groups I've either helped to establish or founded. It's a time of accomplishment.

My love for my husband continues to grow and I do as much as I can to help him as he grows older. We really enjoy each other's company more with each passing year. I'm lucky in that I married the love of my life. He is so good to me and I try to be as good to him.

I've broken my ankle and had a rough several months in recovery, making it hard to do the hard physical labor of gardening a ninety bed organic garden on a fairly steep hillside, in the northeast area of Georgia. But because of my experience, knowledge, and willingness to teach, I have several years of an internship program where I am passing on my knowledge, as well as teaching classes in all that I have learned about growing and preserving food organically, and making my own medicines with herbs I also grow. I consult, mentor, help a lot of people to learn and apply those things which brings me great joy. And I also work with my church to help people achieve greater spiritual strength and freedom.

So, menopause is just a bodily function which is natural to the female of the species, and which then leaves us so that we can concentrate on our greater function of nurturing our tribe, our families, our people with all that we bring to the table from what we have learned.

It's that or sit in front of the television and become stuffed statues of our former selves. It's a choice we can make. I chose to enjoy the heck out of life and go for the relationships with people around me, and learn as much as I can, as well as find ways to pass that on to a society that is falling apart at the seams from stress, a few crazy greedy people who want to change our world into a pile of rubble, and other pressures we had no clue would ever come to us fifty years ago. It's a time when cooler heads who know how to predict how things, will go and work to keep humanity going in the right and survival direction.

If you've lived over fifty years, you see patterns in how things go and can look into the future with some measure of sanity and understanding. I think that is our greatest gift to the younger members of the tribe. And our ability to love them, teach them, give them a hand when they need it, and stand up to the bad decisions at any level of society and work to bring goodness back in. We have that power, us old coots, and we better use it because in a society that has worshiped youth for a long time, with the outcomes as we see them, it's about time we used our power to keep us from blowing ourselves to smithereens or degenerating into a bunch of barbarians. We need civilization and that comes from wisdom and stable people.

Look in the mirror. That's YOU.

Diann Dirks

Six

My grandmothers never talked about menopause. Ever. We all just witnessed sudden and cataclysmic shifts in how our grandmothers approached every day and life in general.

My Grandmother Thomas would just sit staring into the gathering dusk like she really wasn't present or when helping my Grandmother Holder set the table, before a meal, she would grab the silverware out of my hand, scream at me that I was slow as a snail then slam the silverware in place after place by each plate.

Linda Gay Brown

Seven

On Turning Fifty

    1.

My friends and I tell each other,
You're looking good, not adding
what is understood—*for your age*.
Getting ready takes longer now,
with diminishing returns.
We trade lotions and tinctures,
compare sun damage,
discuss when to let our hair go gray.

(Aunt Horty's hair still blazed
at eighty—red as in fire, defiance.
Cigarette in one hand,
gin and tonic in the other,
she joked, *Remember what
the undertaker said—
any day above ground is a good day*.)

    2.

All these years aiming
to please parents, lovers, husbands—
all of whom we disappointed
and who disappointed us in turn
(forgive us our shortcomings)—
we did not see
we were Amazons in the making,
fighting to claim our own stories.

Now is the time of our unbecoming,
to shed the selves
constructed all these years.
Unwind the layers
like gauze around a mummy.
In the heart center an ember glows.
This is where the true self dwells,
She Who Knows.

    3.

How long has it been
since I ran full-throttle, plunged
into the ocean, let the waves
knock me about? Why am I not,
this minute, dancing?
It's time to crank up the music again,
"Burning Down the House."

    4.

I dream myself old
in loose clothes and straw hat,
hoeing a garden, sweeping a porch.
Insects whir, a cat basks nearby.
I move slowly
and do not think of mirrors,
pain, or even God.
As Venus transits the sickle moon,
I breathe in the stillness.
This, I say to no one. *This.*

Debra Kaufman

Eight

Hi, it's Faye from Ontario.

I am sixty-one. And my mom is alive and well at eighty-five. Lucky me. My mom started menopause at forty, and had hot flashes and night sweats to the degree that she would have to get up in the middle of the night and change the sheets. Poor woman. She started hormone therapy at some point and the symptoms eased somewhat but never went away. She actually got cervical cancer in her sixties and my sister and I felt it was because of the hormone therapy. She recovered from the cancer but had to go off the hormone therapy. It was awful again, soaking wet in the night. After two years she got a clean bill of health and she begged the doctor to let her go back on hormone therapy. She did and felt saved again although to this day she has hot flashes.

She lives in Alberta where I was raised and they have Chinooks, that wonderful weather pattern that comes in over the Rockies and suddenly what was once a cold bitter day becomes balmy, no jacket weather. So my mom says "I'm having a Chinook" as she waves her hand in front of her face and turns beet red.

How did that impact me, you might be wondering. Well, when I was about forty I started a mantra, "I will not be like my mother, I will not be like my mother" (just in relation to menopause). I said it often and deliberately because oh my gosh I did not want to live that. IT

WORKED! I actually sailed through menopause, only about a year of a few hot flashes at about age fifty-one. No problemo. My sister, on the other hand, who is seven years younger than me, has hot flash issues. She has tried the patch, gained a bunch of weight and then ripped it off, went to the health food store and got some stuff. It is working so far. She is fifty-four. Drinking red wine seems to set her off though. I found that too. White isn't so bad ... what is all that about?

I must tell you about the celebration I did though. So my friends and I who all went through this together started talking about becoming Crones. Crones in a positive sense. I threw a Crone Party for myself. It was my coming of age for going into menopause. It was a grand affair. We all dressed elegantly and I hired my 25-year-old daughter and friend to make the food and serve us. They were a delight – the young maidens in a crowd of old crones. I sent Tim off somewhere as no men allowed. Two of my friends are puppeteers and they did a performance in my honour. Two large women puppets 'of a certain age,' going through a suitcase of memorabilia, all attached to me and my progression to *cronehood* – if there is such a thing. At one point in the evening I was wearing a crinoline under a beautiful teal blue skirt and dancing like no one was watching. Oh such fun.

I work with many similar-aged women, and we share the camaraderie of hot flashes and forgetfulness...like having to replace a lot of nouns with adjectives in order to arrive at the right noun:

"Oh, you know, the grey chair with the leg thingy that goes up with the thingy on the side…ahhhhhhh…Oh, yeah. The lazy boy chair."

This kind of crazy loss of nouns still goes on quite regularly, unfortunately.

Good luck with everything!

Your friend on the Ontario farm,

Faye Blondin

Nine

Dear Sister,

It was autumn, just as it is now as I write you this letter. From the window of my apartment I can glimpse the sea winking in the golden rays of late afternoon. Autumn: that mellow time when the sun seems to linger forever. But the sun's rays didn't reach into my doctor's surgery. It was a little cool in there, with a sniff of antiseptic in the air, and I could hear the rumble of traffic from the main road outside.

I was forty-two years old and feeling foolish, dear sister. You see, after some years of faltering cycles, I hadn't bled for twelve months. But it wasn't till this day that I told my doctor. She looked me in the eye and said, "It looks like you've gone through menopause."

My first reaction was complete surprise. Then I felt elated. Wow! I'd had a super-easy menopause: just a gradual withdrawal of the flow, with a few nights when it seemed that I might have had some mild hot flushes. No other symptoms. No more bleeding, no more contraception. Fantastic!

But then, as I walked out of the doctor's rooms, the smile soon left my eyes. I wandered home, curled up on my favourite window seat in the sun, and wept. No more babies, no more fertility. Even though I didn't want any more, the finality of menopause hit me hard.

Who was I now? Some of my friends were still getting pregnant. Would people laugh at me, treat me differently if I said I was post-menopausal?

Three years later, I gathered together all the post-menopausal women I could find. I ran workshops with the aim of creating an art project about menopause. I dug for the good news and created a celebration called 'Threshold' that included story-telling, poems, a book called 'Crone-ologies,' music and a collaborative installation.

The response from other women was fantastic. We felt wild and powerful. I had now become so defiant that I purchased a number plate for my Mitsubishi Mirage car that said CRONE and drove it around town laughing at people's reactions. My mother, who never spoke about such things, was dismayed and embarrassed by my behaviour. But later she told me that she'd had a terrible menopause, and had endured heavy bleeding for years rather than agree to a hysterectomy.

There was another consequence that I had not anticipated. Osteoporosis runs in the family, and within a decade of menopause a scan revealed that my bone density had dropped alarmingly. It's taken twenty years trying different medications before I've finally stopped the bone loss. (I discovered Algaecal's plant-based calcium, and Strontium Plus, a natural remedy that is now building new bone.)

Looking back, I realise I made a mistake. When my periods

started slowing down in my late thirties, a naturopath put me on a herbal mixture that restored the flow. But after some time on this remedy, in my youthful arrogance, I decided to stop it and 'let nature decide.' Nature did decide, and it wasn't the best thing. I wish now that I'd been able to keep my cycle going, even if only for another five years.

The ancient wisdom talks of menopause as a time when we hold the wise blood inside. I'm wiser now, and thankfully my bones are recovering. I wish I'd been wiser all those years ago.

Love from Auckland, New Zealand,

Juliet Batten

Ten

There is more to menopause than hot flashes and night sweats. There is insomnia, anxiety, heart palpitations and so much more. But it really is no big deal. This too shall pass and in the meantime there are fewer cramps, less PMS and less money spent on tampons. It all evens out and really, we can't avoid it so just go with the flow, or away from the flow. Ha!

Amanda King

Eleven

I too have no mother or grandmothers to look to for guidance. When I was in my late thirties my aunt offered me a very sad looking 'what to expect' book and I said no thanks — something, anything than that to better shed light and wisdom on menopause. My issue has been dissuading bloody doctors since I turned forty that everything is about perimenopause and to just suck it up.

Don't be too sure you're on the road to menopause. Doctors are people too, and even professionals can assume, project, be misinformed or not up-to-date. Your birth-date isn't the only indicator once you hit your forties.

Just a few months shy of forty I needed contraception again and was prescribed the mini-pill, the doctor assuring me that my age and that of my partner, almost fifty, meant we had a much lesser risk of falling pregnant as I was likely in peri-menopause. A few months later, her advice proved wrong. Several of my school friends also had pregnancies and children in their forties, one at forty-eight.

At forty-three, I experienced irregular menstrual cycles, mood swings and tiredness. The doctor did a blood test, looked at my birth-date and sent me away from the ten minute appointment with the words peri-menopause ringing in my ears. I wasn't in the mood to go into menopause without a fight, so I went to a Chinese Herbalist who actually read the blood test results, noting elevated liver enzyme and cholesterol readings. After two hours of questions she said my qi (energy) was unbalanced. After six months of drinking her vile tasting herbal tea concoctions, and twice weekly, weekly, fortnightly, then monthly visits – all was back to normal.

Just after my forty-fifth birthday I started to feel tired, have to have a nap on the sofa after work tired. I put it down to the effects of the end of a very busy work project. I took several weeks holiday over Christmas & New Year and returned still tired. I was having trouble mustering the energy to get out of bed so my partner made the sensible suggestion I go to the doctor. As I chronicled my symptoms and circumstances to her I mentioned a work colleague had glandular fever a few months back, and my younger sister over Christmas had been ill with possible Glandular Fever but not confirmed. The doctor consulted my birth-date and proffered the opinion that it was a virus that affects younger people, not the over-forties. I insisted on the blood test anyway. The blood test results confirmed it – I had glandular fever, and the same later for my sister.

At forty-seven, my menstrual cycle became irregular again. I thought, ok, this is it, peri-menopause. I didn't bother going to the doctor but searched via the Internet for suggestions and came up with quite a few results regarding the necessity of Vitamin D for reproductive health. I work 9-5 weekdays in an office, and at that time adhered to the slip-slop-slap sunscreen, sunglasses, sleeves, hat regime when in sunlight. After moderating my slip-slop-slap behaviours, getting some sun and taking a good Vitamin D + Calcium supplement, over a year later my menstrual cycle is still what is considered regular. I am forty-eight, living in Sydney Australia, and it's not that I think I can avoid menopause – I simply want to be properly informed and deal with what's real.

Ella Dee

Twelve

Dear Little Sister (that I never had),

Growing up in Ohio as the youngest of four children I grew up in the knowledge that being a young girl and growing into a woman was something that was pretty special. I possessed qualities that the guys in my family just didn't have nor would they ever have. I also grew up thinking that I would have very similar experiences as my mother and my sister when it came to childbirth and that dreaded menopause experience. I was wrong. Life is funny that way when we go into it with certain expectations.

Let me clarify things a bit. I am not in menopause. To be officially in menopause Aunt Flo needs to have not visited me for twelve months. Just when I think that that is going to be the case she shows up on my doorstep with her suitcase in hand. I am almost fifty-four and *I* think I should be far past this phase of my life but sadly I am not.

So I suspect I am among those who are lingering in the peri-menopause chapter of life and not really happy about it. I just want to get on with it. Move on. Get over it. Enough already. I am tired of always packing my little *supplies* when we travel on the off chance that Aunt Flo decides to arrive unexpectedly at our destination.

I am tired of sleepless nights. I am tired of flipping and flopping trying to get some shut eye. I am tired of refluffing my pillows multiple times a night in the effort to get some quality sleep. Let's face it…I am tired.

I am tired of having my husband refer to me as "a hunk of burning love" because when he touches me at night my skin is on fire. I am tired of being the glowing nightlight at night. And then, just as soon as it starts it disappears and I need to bury myself in covers to get warm again. It is unpredictable. That is probably the worst part of this lovely time of peri-menopause is the unpredictability of it all. If it was predictable I believe it would be a tad bit easier to deal with the changes that my body is experiencing.

Those changes include and are not limited to: weight gain, mood changes, changes in sexual desires and needs, and changes in bone density and cholesterol numbers. Look what you have to look forward to! It is a bit overwhelming when I think about it. There is a lot going on in my body and it is not always fun. But it is part of being a woman and try as I might I cannot imagine that I would be happy being anything other than the woman that I am.

Why do I think it is all worth it? Because it allowed me to be a mom. Being a mom is without a doubt the best job I have ever had in my entire life. It has brought me much happiness and joy. When I look at my adult sons and realize that a part of me is actually in them it makes me smile and I am amazed at how something like that happens. How on earth does this all transpire? How do we put a man and woman together and create such amazing people?

On those days when I feel like a frumpy almost-54-year-old I check my battle scars—the scar from one C-section, the not so taut tummy, the wrinkles that are now appearing on my face and I remember that with the wonderful things often come the not so wonderful things. In order to be able to be a mom I have to experience all phases of life and it somehow puts it all into a bit of perspective. I can choose to dwell on the negatives of being a woman and the inevitable menopause and all that it brings with it or I can choose to focus on the positives.

The positives are often right in front of me. The obvious joy that I possess because I am a mom. While I know that this is not the path that all women want or can even achieve for various reasons…for me it is the best positive that I can put my finger on. It has brought me joy beyond measure and continues to bring me added joy with each new accomplishment that they achieve as adults. I continue to nurture them from afar and am a cheerleader.

The very things that make me a woman are the positives in my life. My ability to be compassionate and nurturing, to see the good in others and to promote positive things in this world are there right before me. What a wonderful gift it is to be able to identify these as the joys of being a woman in her fifties and to embrace them. That, to me, is what it is all about. Embracing the goodness that we all have and can share. Even in the peri-menopause season of my life I can see that I have things to offer others that are unique to my experience of being a woman.

Change is not always bad, and as I step back and look at the changes that are occurring as a result of being a woman I am finding that change can be good. After all—this is simply a season of my life. It will pass, eventually, and it is a necessity before I reach the next stage.

I am fifty-three. My advice is to embrace it. Make jokes about your hot flashes and night sweats. Roll with the punches. Accept that there are going to be some days that you are going to go into a full out crying jag when one of those sad "save the animals" commercials comes on television. Embrace those days when your pants fit. Cherish one more hug from a child. When it is all said and done you are a woman, and quite honestly—that is the best thing to be.

Beth Ann Chiles

Thirteen

Dear Cecilia's little Sister,

I'm forty-nine now, live in Portland, Oregon and I stopped having my period almost three years ago.

I was peri-menopausal for years; which means I had body odor, mood swings and night sweats yet still had the good fortune to get my period! After more than five years enjoying sweating through my pajamas in the middle of the winter and slamming my car door so hard in a tantrum over forgetting the dry cleaning that now the car window rattles if it isn't all the way rolled up…after five years of that, I got to menopause. My naturally oily skin and hair isn't so oily anymore which is really great because I don't have to shampoo my hair everyday if I don't want to. I also look younger than my years. My acne keeps me looking youthful.

That's right! There is another bonus to menopause (NOT another one Maggie! Our middle-aged woman cup over-floweth!) Oh, yeah, I thought the zits were gone for good but they're not. Nope, they are back and they are cystically new and improved. Old age acne is different than the acne I remember from back in the glory days of tetracycline and BufPufs. Now I get bumps that I think will be zits but nothing really happens. The bump appears, gets really big and red and noticeable; then after a month or so dies down and goes away.

I have a whisker on my chin. Just one wiry whisker that showed up in the past year. I tweeze it as soon as I feel it poking out from my jaw line. Great.

I have days when I can sense a hormonal funk coming on. Ahhhh....hormones. Life issues like concern over one of my kid's grades or wanting a new couch are not taken in stride. On hormone days, I quickly go from teary to bitter to angry to barely controlled, seething rage and finally collapsing into hopelessly fat. And I run that gamut of emotions in about ninety seconds.

Everyone is different. I don't think there is a set of menopause symptoms or side effects that everyone gets. But, I do think anything strange that is new to you is most likely due to hormones. If you feel like a furnace just turned on in your uterus, probably hormones. If you start crying because no one asked what your New Year's resolution is, it's probably hormones. If you stop drinking wine for a month and don't lose an ounce, it's probably hormones. Drink water and lots of wine and talk to your friends, they are most likely feelin' it too!

Maggie O'Connor

Fourteen

When my period stopped at age forty-three, it was the happiest day of my life. Bar none.

Menarche started for me at age eleven, and every month brought a week or more of excruciating pain with other symptoms such as excessive bleeding, clots, vomiting and diarrhea. I saw many doctors over the years who performed D&Cs, cauterizations, gave me hormones and other drugs. I saw naturopaths and acupuncturists. I got massage, exercised and watched my diet. Nothing made much difference.

Menopause was like being released from prison. No more scalding hot baths. No more ruining my clothes. Kicking off my covers at night was a privilege compared to the previous thirty-two years of suffering.

Menopause was heaven. I highly recommend it.

Love from Marshalltown, Iowa,

Sandy Wyatt

Fifteen

I remember the summer of 1978 like it was yesterday. Huddled on the floor in the back corner of the Southwest Branch Library, clutching a copy of *Are You There, God? It's Me, Margaret* in my trembling eleven-year-old hands.

Six months after Mom's death, and I didn't know what was happening to me. Had I done something terrible that had caused the bleeding? Was *I* going to die soon, too? Doctors weren't my friends — after all, they weren't able to keep Momma alive, so there was *no way* I was going to trust them with *this* terrible discovery. There was no way I was going to tell Daddy, either. He didn't understand these things and would take me right to them. I was sure of it.

Thirty-six years later, I find myself in much the same situation — sneaking in moments on the laptop, frantically typing in "symptoms of perimenopause." Hoping for an answer. Hoping that someone will tell me these horribly unpredictable physical and emotional spikes I'm having are just part of the "change of life" — whatever *that* means. Hoping that the 3am panic attacks, huddled on the bathroom floor, will be over soon. Hoping that my husband doesn't secretly think I'm a frigid, emotional bitch and that he'll still be there with me when this has ended.

The female rites of passage I've had to experience so far have been a solo journey — no Wise Woman at my side, helping to soothe the monthly dread of having to "dress out" for junior high gym class. To tell me about what having sex for the first time would feel like. To lend a shoulder of support when the doctor said a hysterectomy was highly recommended because my 38-year-old uterus was filled with tumors that had probably been growing there for some time.

Where are my Grandmothers? Where are the gatherings of women who have braved the passage and are willing to teach? Where are my sisters, who also prepare to venture into this unknown territory?

I am a woman, trapped and shaking, in a little girl's body. Huddled in the corner, all over again, hoping that the next page in the book will reveal all the Great Mysteries.

"Are you there, Goddess? It's me, Leigh."

Leigh Tyler Olsen

Sixteen

Life is a journey unto self.

> "Life is brief, it takes courage to live deep."
> — Anonymous

We live in a sunburnt country. Mostly we have heat and dry. But after the rain the smell of eucalyptus heavily scents the air. It is far away from growing up in the farmlands of Southern Ohio. A chance meeting with the love of my life brought me to remote Australia, thirty years ago. I left my family and friends to live in a country I'd never laid eyes on. It was before the Internet and email. Telephone calls were expensive, a letter took two weeks by air mail. The stagecoach only visited once a month. Just kidding about the stagecoach.

Through mutual effort I maintained close contact with the important women in my life. I am blessed to have very close female relationships, especially with my mother. Helpful though that was, in the years building to menopause, I can tell you, my journey was different to theirs. And chances are, yours will be different to most of the women you know too. There are similarities, but it seems to me, everyone's experience is a result of the mysterious cocktail of genetics and their ability to live deeper. Peeling away the layers and going deeply into yourself – finding what you are made of – that is the real journey.

- Embrace the changes Life brings. Read, take courses, start a new hobby, eat new foods, meet new people, renew yourself. (Recommended reading: Sarah Ban Breathnach's. *Simple Abundance* and the blog bemorewithless.com)
- Our bodies are the vehicle for our souls on this earth. They need a 'tune up' now and then.
- Ask… Receive… Be grateful. Help doesn't always come from whom you expect. I learned to ask for help, receive it gratefully, and in turn, how to offer it.
- Good energy attracts good energy. Our thoughts, words and deeds are all energy, which contribute to our wellbeing. This does not mean bad or uncomfortable things will not happen if we think good thoughts; it just helps the journey be more gratifying.
- Everything is easier if you are not sleep deprived. Night sweats made me appreciate a good night's sleep! Make sleep a priority.
- At the age of sixty I bless every day I don't have cramps, heavy bleeding or a migraine, which is every day now!
- My uterus and ovaries (not to mention my husband) gave us our daughter, the most precious blessing of my life. They were there when it mattered, and I am grateful. I don't have them (still have the husband!) now, and I'm grateful for that too!
- If your daughter is going through puberty at the same time you are mid-journey to menopause, *see previous point* for frequent reminding about 'said blessing.'
- Become your own advocate. It beats every career

choice I ever made. Read, educate yourself, talk to loved ones, but make your OWN decisions. (Read *Women's Bodies, Women's Wisdom* and *The Wisdom of Menopause*, both by Christiane Northrup.)
• Breast cancer and the challenges with Menopause have enriched my life immeasurably because I did not simply *endure* them; I was led by them to discover a deeper self. No do-overs necessary.

Listen… to your body… to your inner voice. Examine patterns and frustrations for learning opportunities. Nurture yourself with good food, good people and take time for YOU. In sacrificing yourself for others, you risk losing your Self. Be kind and nurturing, of course, but do that for yourself, as well as others. To my dear, young-adult daughter I say, *Be kind to yourself.*

Talk to yourself with the love and care you would show a small child. That small child still lives inside you…a revealing journey away, but still there.

Hugs and more hugs (because every good journey should end with a hug),

Ardys Zoellne

Seventeen

Dear sister,

As a preteen, bras, breasts, and menstruation – and the lack of them – obsessed me. I started kindergarten at four, so I was a year younger than everyone in my grade. By eighth grade, my girlfriends not only had breasts and were wearing bras, adding insult to injury, they had periods to boot. I was so envious. No one had explained to me that because I was a year younger, I would start later, and I was too dumb to figure it out on my own. And even if anyone *had* explained things to me, no one could ever accuse me of having an optimistic, laid-back disposition. Inconsolable, I was always begging for a brassiere even though, regrettably, I didn't need one. Always pouring over ads for Kotex in *American Girl* Magazine that asked, "Are You in the Know?"

So the moment I did have my first period on October 12th, 1954 (I was thirteen and in my freshman year in high school), I was ecstatic. I bolted out of the bathroom and announced my 'discovery' to my mother. Her voice dripped with sarcasm. "*Well, con-gra-tu-la-tions!*" She was forty-three at the time and perhaps she was going through *her* menopause.

Tampax was a new product, at least to me. (I have today learned via the Internet tampons have been around forever and Tampax since 1936. Who knew?) So I toddled right up to the drugstore and bought some. When my mother discovered that sea-blue package in the bathroom closet, she went ballistic and dragged me 'by the ear' to the doctor to make sure I was still a virgin; she stood next to the doctor during the examination.

Over the years, strange as it may sound, I loved having a period, even though I recall spending some days in bed with a heating pad. It made me feel womanly. When menopause came along, I don't know why but I did not suffer night sweats or flushing and had no physical symptoms per se. My personality was another thing. I have always been a prickly, super-sensitive person, and menopause certainly didn't improve me, but neither would you much have noticed.

When my periods tapered off in my early fifties, instead of being grateful and gleeful, I would sob with relief at my surprise visit: Yes! One more time! I was still a vibrant woman, still in the game, so to speak. I'm seventy-three now, I live in Chicago and though I'm well out of it, I don't *feel* out of it. This to me is the most amazing fact of all. I haven't lost my libido yet. And after all, this is what, for me, it's always been about.

Anonymous

Eighteen

I was the last child of my generation — with much older cousins and aunts, and a mother that was disinterested, a product of her times. So I don't have any old wisdom that has been carefully handed down, only my own experiences. That could make me a 'primary source' as research would call it — but in science, the validity of the project requires repetition of the same result. I am only one — and am not going to volunteer to re-experience the whole thing again. Time travel being so complicated.

My mother's generation, being very proper, did not discuss 'bodily functions.' She would not even say "toilet paper" in public or write it out on a grocery list — which ended up in odd purchases if my dad or I picked up the groceries. While living a generally healthy life, I do know she bled heavily for three months until the doctor performed 'The Operation.' Every ache, pain, pound gained, difficulty after that was blamed on 'The Operation.'

As I got older, I figured what was going to happen would happen. Pioneer women on the frontier lived through it and survived. So I just glanced at articles and research that appeared, gathered authoritative background knowledge, and shrugged.

Letters for my Little Sister

No use worrying. It's like running a medical trial. If you tell test subjects what they can expect to experience, that's what they report experiencing.

Still you hear all those whispers from talk shows, neighbors, magazine articles written by celebrities-who-know-it-all, and normal looking people who are selling a book they wrote. Constant nagging-warning-worry-inciting-terror whispers. Swatting all that away like flies, you just keep climbing that mountain of age – expecting a great cliff and deep chasm anytime. Trudging on with determination to withstand the worst when it comes.

When one day you notice the whispers have stopped. You look around and realize you passed that feared end-of-life-as-you-know-it cliff long ago. All that is ahead are clear skies and green valleys to enjoy (you can insert your own image of rainbows and unicorns and such here).

Those years weren't totally free of annoying issues, but I didn't even recognize when menopause started. (Life was busy.) Periods that had been long and heavy gradually became a day shorter, then another day shorter. So much lighter. Then hardly there. Was it a cosmic joke or a big welcome when the last time 'my friend' (as Mother called it) came to visit for half a day end of December, 1999?

Over. Done. Hasn't made much difference. Although I can't eat whenever, whatever, and as much as I want any more. Doctors say not to get too thin – you need a bit of padding as you age. (Fine, but not so much there, please.) Oh, the treadmill twenty minutes a day to maintain weight, or forty minutes to take off weight. It does work... so you can still eat ice cream.

One bit of warning. Do not let yourself, family, or doctors blame everything on 'change of life.' It's so easy to do that. If there's a health issue ask "Just for fun, what else could this be?" I was lucky. An astute doctor looked at me and said, "This could be menopause-related, but it could be something else." There seems to be an epidemic of middle-aged women with thyroid disruption. They don't know why, yet. After forty-eight hours on medication, I no longer felt drained, and exhausted — dead. I never even realized I felt so bad. You just expect that as you get older? Don't settle!

Other advice? Wear cotton or wicking clothing for night sweats. Disrupted sleep was not pleasant. Start exercising now. Walk. Get outdoors in the sunshine at least fifteen minutes a day. (Maria Montessori was right: outside! for all ages!) Eat sensibly. I tried eliminating various 'triggers' and it made no difference at all. Fresh veggies, if possible. An apple, a banana and oatmeal every day will make a difference. Protein is needed. Twice a day take six hundred units of Calcium along with four hundred units of Vitamin D3. And wear shoes. You will kick something and break a toe. You will. Everyone warns and no one listens. Toes never heal right and the shoes you love won't fit. Shoes! (Crocs may look silly, but they are great indoor bumpers for toes.)

One elderly aunt in her nineties once advised, "Just enjoy where you are. Retirement home or assisted living, it's enough for this time of life. Take naps. Get flowers planted by the window. And play Bingo. Always. You never know who's going to have a funny story. Sometimes you win. If you don't, there's always the next game. Bingo is good."

So there you have it. Just smile. Keep going. Be informed but consider the source. Take care of yourself the best you can. And Bingo.

There are seagulls calling overhead as they fly from the wetlands to the coast.

I am sixty-five this year. Older than you, but not old.

From the shores of Clear Lake Texas,

Karen W. Parker

Nineteen

Journal entries during this time in my life

> 5/26 [after a conflict with my husband]. I feel like everything is a test, is symbolic of something bigger, that I've failed in some way. Just by being who I am, I'm inadequate, not "fun," that what interests me—reading, writing, yoga, solitude—makes me boring. I've written about this before. It should be OK. *I should be OK.* Why do I feel like the female dog on her back, throat open, belly open, the submissive "don't hurt me" pose. Afraid to claim my power. Not even aware what "power" means. To me it just means being true to yourself. Why should this be hard? Fuck it, life's too short. My soul wants to be free to express herself.
>
> Evelyn said once that she saw me as an angel with one wing pinned behind my back. Let her go, let her flap both heavy feathered wings, let them unfurl, shake out the dust and debris, let the fresh air billow them like sails. Don't deny that transformation is occurring; that as middle age, with its mockery of the body, accumulates, the soul is wanting to move toward the light, toward a deeper beauty. Do not be mired in the muck of petty concerns. Fly upwards but don't forget about earth. Be aware and part of earth and its richness without getting ground down by it, have a larger vision, be mindful of it, don't waste energy on ego, hurt feelings, someone projecting their stuff onto you.

Debra Kaufman

Twenty

Now that I'm actually through the whole process I can rejoice and say YIPPEE! But the beginning and the process of Menopause was completely miserable.

My grandmother and my mother and therefore, I, all started going through peri-menopause in our late thirties. My grandmother was a true southern lady, she NEVER talked about the problems 'the change' was causing her. My mother was a very progressive woman; she was extremely open about what was happening to her body. As for both of them and myself the worst, the absolutely worst was the extreme feeling of heat – night sweats so bad the sheets and the night gown had to be changed, sometimes three or more times a night. Hot flashes that could happen in an instant without any prior warning. One minute you feel comfortable, the next sweat is pouring off of you. Just sitting down to get a haircut and having the cosmetologist place a cape around your neck and shoulders could and would set off a hot flash.
For the three of us – Gram, Mom and myself – (my three daughters are not experiencing any of this) the heat flashes were the worst.

Some of my friends experienced painful intercourse, foggy or spacey feelings and memories, anxiety, and worry about getting old.

Nope, not us. It was being hot…all the time…way too hot. So hot just the thought of a blanket on you at night would set off a major chain reaction of sweating, changing the bed sheets and showering to don a clean set of night clothes.

Even as my Mother moved into her late sixties I could still see her sitting outside on her patio trying to cool down as the sweat poured off her face.

Today I am in my middle sixties and I too have the same affliction. All I have to do is get a little concerned or alarmed over something…not much….too much thinking about things I need to do the next day will set the heat off. But!!! Hallelujah…it is Nothing compared to ten years ago!

My mother passed on her seventieth birthday, so I'm thinking that I will get to find out what the seventies bring since she isn't here to tell me.

Oh, yes…you get really dry 'down there'…that is miserable also. I really don't have an answer for how to move through any of this or what to do for it. I guess just take one day at a time and be grateful for that day. And if you really want to, your physician can provide estrogen cream to ease things.

Linda Gay Brown

Twenty-One

Dear Celi's Little Sister,

This is the story of the menopause that wasn't. I pray you'll never have to go through anything like this. Hope for a normal one, warts and all…

In December 2011, I was fifty-one years old, single, and in good health. I was a normal weight for my height, I ate a good, healthy diet and life was more or less OK, except for losing my job the previous month. On December 23rd, I received a diagnosis of breast cancer. Happy Christmas to me. It shouldn't have come as a surprise; we have an overpowering history of it in our family's women. I was on my own, all my family was far away. I just had to get on with it. In a way, I was taking the statistical hit for my sisters, and was grateful they didn't have to go through it too.

After surgery in January and February 2012, chemo started in March. Blood tests before it started showed I was nowhere near menopause, so the chemo for my 100% ER/PR (estrogen/progesterone) positive cancer was tailored to shut down hormone production to help prevent its return. The chemo itself was pretty horrible. I still don't know how much of the sleeplessness, hot sweats, restlessness and chemo-brain fog were the anti-cancer drugs, and how much of it was a side effect of having all female hormone production in my body brought to a screeching halt in a matter of a few days. Whatever the cause, the effect was severe. And as it turned out, lasting.

Sometimes the body comes back from the chemical assault. If you're young enough, and your hormones are still in full swing. I wasn't, and mine weren't. Not menopausal, just not in my female prime any longer. By the time chemo was over, so were my hormones. And now I take Tamoxifen to try and convince any remaining cancer cells that there's nothing here for them. That has its own charming set of side effects ...

For me, the most distressing side effect of menopause has been the weight gain. Some of it was due to the steroids you take while on chemo. Post cancer, post menopausal weight gain is the hardest to lose. Your body isn't producing hormones from the normal sources. So other parts of you step up to fill the demand. Notably adipose (fatty) tissue, which has the capability to produce small amounts of female hormones. The less hormones you have, the more the body tells itself it needs fat to make more hormones, the more fat you tend to gain.

If oncologists were completely candid about the side effects of chemotherapy, many women would refuse it. I wasn't especially lucky; a lot of it hit me harder than other women. And I think if I had to do it again to live, I would, but I'd be better prepared this time. But I definitely don't want to go through menopause again: hot flushes, poor sleep, poor memory for words and names, dry skin and eyes, weight gain (two dress sizes), a flare-up in my arthritis.

I have no idea how long I can expect it to go on; my mother and two of my older sisters had hysterectomies before they reached menopause. One other sister has gone through it, and sailed through without trouble. I'd say the hot flushes were the most disabling: some nights the bedclothes are off and on like a tart's knickers! But I tell myself it's a small price to pay in return for the rest of my life. Of course, if the cancer comes back, I'm going to be extremely grumpy…

Still forgetful, frequently tired and often sweaty.

Love from Queensland, Australia,

Kate Chiconi

Twenty-Two

I'm not exactly sure when it started, but it was earlier than I expected it to happen. I was in my late thirties when I started having night sweats. I just thought I was hot. I did live in south Texas, after all. I would turn one hundred and eighty degrees in the bed so that my head was under the ceiling fan to be cooler. My husband thought I was a bit mad. I realized eventually that this was the beginning of the beguine, the slow dance to the quieting of the reproductive system. I had no problem with menopause — I just wished it would hurry up and be over.

I had no idea what it would be like for me. I don't know if my mother had started menopause before she died at the age of fifty-two. She was forty-two when first diagnosed with breast cancer. I am an only child and I was still in high school. At the time, I was very self involved and discovering alcohol, drugs, and boys, in that order. We never discussed her pain or what was happening with her body. She had surgery, she recovered, she moved on. The cancer came back five years later in the other breast and then again five years later in the brain, lungs, and liver and she was gone. She was both fragile and strong. The youngest of four, my mother was born in 1937 and grew up on my grandfather's one hundred acre cotton farm. She contracted polio as a child and survived with the help of her mother and sisters, but she never spoke of it. After she died, I learned more about my mother from her sisters than I ever knew about her when she was alive.

There has always been a fear in the back of my mind of breast cancer, that it would happen to me too, but it hasn't so far. For that, I am grateful. My doctor has informed me that the odds of having breast cancer decrease very significantly after menopause, so that is a great thing. Something to do with hormone levels. But then again, another doctor told me that the symptoms of menopause could last ten years before everything was over. Great, I thought at the time, time to get a bigger air conditioner. As it turns out, it did last for about ten years, in varying degrees of intensity.

My periods were always regular, birth control pills are good for that, but even after I had my tubes tied, they were regular. I have wondered if my symptoms were better or worse because I had no children. I don't know. But I didn't want children and neither did my husband. The periods just came less frequently and finally stopped. I did have hot flashes, but they weren't bad, just occasional and no perspiration, just a flushed, red-faced feeling that would go away in a few minutes.

The absolute worst thing for me was the mood swings. My emotions can be mercurial as it is and the hormonal changes did not help. Many times, it felt like I had been turned up to eleven… not one louder, but one crazier. It was really bad for a couple of years. My rage was ever present or I was depressed/despondent or I was paralyzed with terror. I never knew where I would be on the spectrum and neither did my husband. Stress at work or at home only made it worse. I had no coping skills. However, exercise helped tremendously. I wish I had been more consistent about the exercise. I would have had an easier time of it, I think. When I was walking consistently, I felt better emotionally and the hot flashes abated. I am a recovering alcoholic and drug addict, but I was so desperate that I even tried pot again after twenty years. It didn't help. My husband and I smoked the same amount from the same joint. He was mellow and goofy. For me, every muscle in my body tensed up and I was bitchy, make that bitchy-er. Epic fail, dude, epic fail. It might work for some women though. That is just my experience.

My body is different. My skin is a lot drier. I inherited my mother's oily skin which has helped me in the wrinkle department, but was always annoying in the grease factor department. But now it is not as oily and can even be dry if the weather is not very humid. I use a lot of moisturizer in the mornings and have started applying moisturizer at night as well after I have washed my face. I often feel like one of those women in the movies from the 1950's and 60's. Do you remember those? She would be sitting at her make-up table in front of the mirror applying creams to her face and neck. I always thought that was so elegant. I do that now, only in shorts and a t-shirt, not in an elegant gown. I have no lighted make up table, so I just sit on the edge of the bed and talk to the cats about their day as I apply creams. The cats often comment on the smoothness of my skin after I have finished. However, they could just want some cat treats…sneaky cats.

I started getting dark hairs on my chin when all of this started and it has only gotten worse…more dark hairs…. UGH! I have a high powered lighted magnifying mirror to keep up with them. I even started getting dark hairs on my neck. I remain on the lookout. I will not embrace the dark hairs as part of my womanhood. It's not happening.

Sex. I don't have much desire, but my husband doesn't either, so we match in that respect. I know how lucky I am. There is still a lot of cuddling though and handholding. Honestly, if there is a quota on sexual activity, I think I met mine by the time I was in my mid thirties. I was a bit of a hussy. It's kind of a relief.

My hair is not as thick as it used to be, which saddens me, but I keep it short. It's cooler. I am not going bald or anything. There is just less hair. It covers my head and that is fine. I still perspire at night unless it's chilly outside, but not as badly as before. That may never change, I don't know.

One major change I have made that has helped so much: I noticed that I was losing muscle tone at an alarming rate and had gained quite a few pounds during the 'menopause years.' I joined a gym this last summer to regain some muscle mass and lose some of the weight. So far, I have lost fifty-five pounds and look better than I have in years. I feel so much better, which is the most important. I have decided that I want to stay strong and keep my bones healthy. Eating right and keeping active works for me. I will do it as long as I can. Life is good at fifty!

Kim

Twenty-Three

A LIFE IN TWO

My mother never taught me much about being a woman. She wanted and perhaps needed a 'best friend' more than daughters, of which she had four. Yet this ally was not someone with whom she could unburden herself, in fact her communication style in general was quite dissimilar to the way close companions and I shared confidences later on in life. She wanted, I think more than anything, to recapture youth lost to The Great Depression coupled with the loss of her own beloved mother; needed relief from a turbulent marriage and motherhood times seven. Mom was a highly creative, intelligent, complicated woman. She died last year at eighty-nine, and I feel as though I never knew her. She was unwilling and perhaps incapable of 'getting real' in the way my generation demanded, and though she doubtlessly loved me, I also made her quite uneasy at times. Numerous queries about everything female, from menses to menopause were answered in the first person clinical, just like the replies she, herself offered doctors in her final years:

> How are you feeling, Mrs. Bowden?
> *Pain, I have pain.* (Gestures absentmindedly with twisted lily hands, blue veins bulging under translucent surface), *All over.*
> What does the pain feel like?
> *Oh, it's neuritis; neuralgia.*
> Forget for a moment what to call it, Mrs. Bowden,

what does the pain feel like? Is it sharp? Dull? Is it twisting, shooting, surging?
It just hurts. All over.

I am not conflicted about the truth in her statements. Build up a lifetime backlog of emotional residue, and a person is bound to suffer. Only two days before she gasped her last precious breath, the hospice doc was still insisting she was physically okay for her age. I did not find this paradox beyond belief.

My mother was a registered nurse who looked up to male doctors (she only went to male doctors, save the woman who delivered me) as though they were gods. Come to think of it, she was a *bona fide* daughter of the Patriarchy. Mom mostly went to physicians to refill the little blue pills *The Stones* termed *mother's little helpers*, getting her through, I suppose, an abusive marriage and the liberation of her offspring out and into the world. What these little azure accomplices also bestowed was a blessed respite from having to engage life on its own terms. Instead she pored over movie magazines, learning more about *the stars* than she did about her own children or, perhaps more importantly, about herself.

I remember the *tête-à-tête* Mom had with me with regards to my first impending period. She was refinishing a set of wooden Windsor chairs in a black lacquer finish, and I can still smell the stain; still envision one of those seats perched atop newspapers spread over the Formica kitchen table. Dad entered the room as she was having 'the talk,' and my stomach clenched as it always did when he stormed about searching for an alcoholic refill. She insisted he leave, and to my amazement no display of histrionics ensued. He simply walked out.

That first menses arrived quite unexpectedly on a seventh-grade class outing to Disneyland, of all places. Clad in white bell-bottom slacks and dreaming of kissing boys on shadowy rides, I got a bulky sanitary napkin from a friend, bought a belt from a machine with a borrowed quarter and wedged the thing into blood-soaked underwear. Tying a sweater around my waist, nobody was the wiser that day, and I did see some kissing action, after all.

Forty years, two marriages and two daughters later, I began bleeding again, this time quite in earnest. Before that, periods were regular, painless two day affairs with a two day trickle-down. This time the bleeding would not stop. I was an exhausted single mother of college-aged young women, engaged in a full-time practice as a Medical Intuitive with several years of radio and column writing to my credit. *Doing it all* was something to which women of my generation were conditioned, perhaps as a backlash to our 'forties and 'fifties frustrated stay-at-home wartime moms.

It did not occur to me to call my mother or my sisters either, come to think of it. Two had gone through menopause in their early forties, I knew that much. I had not spoken to the eldest sister for most of our lives. Though cordially loving when we gathered every few years, we never really knew one another well. Like many fearful households ruled by heavy-handed parents, we were pressured into keeping dark secrets. We were also raised as obedient Mormon women in a decidedly non-Mormon household.

Searching for answers to my dilemma did not lead me down well-travelled roads. I never favored Western medicine beyond its usefulness in acute care. Mom looked to doctors far too much, whereas I was always uncomfortable with their prodding. The invasive questions and cold tools, waiting rooms permeated with apprehension, well-thumbed magazines and sterile, unimaginative surroundings offended my aesthetic sensibilities. It was Mom and her docs who put me on diet pills in junior high just as my body began developing curves. I was not fat, though like my other sisters, subsequently developed a long history of eating disorders.

Females in my family have been labeled a bit high-strung, a bulls-eye target for flustered old-school medical men peddling easy solutions to good-girl patients. Like my mother, her eldest girl child sought after medical opinions and cures, suffering to this day with a host of painful afflictions including Chronic Fatigue and Multiple Sclerosis. Two other sisters have gone on and off Hormone Replacement Therapy (HRT in these days of acronyms) trying, I suppose, to tame the wild woman trapped inside the rules of their religion. I am the only one of four daughters who fled city life and creed in my late teens to embrace the intelligence of trees, of earth and sea and skies. I am the only sister who completed the journey into higher education. Despite our differences, we've all experienced hot flashes well into our sixties.

II

Casting back, I credit that perimenopausal crisis as a life-changing event that continues to infuse my elder years with insight and wisdom. Despite the challenges in learning to balance a body-in-transition, I wouldn't change a thing. During that time of ceaseless bleeding, my eldest was immersed in her Masters Degree in Traditional Chinese Medicine. She introduced me to a particular faculty member at Five Branches University in Santa Cruz, California where she now teaches. Ironically it was this gentle man from Beijing, Yanzhong "Kevin" Zhu, who became my menopause mentor. Trusting he will forgive any misinterpretation on my part, here is my takeaway:

> *Our bodies are of the earth. Right now in these times, humans have appropriated far too much from the planet's core in the way of oil, gas, and so forth. We mine these fossil fuels and then burn them, contributing to a dangerous heating up of the earth's surface. Think of your hot flashes in the same way — you have been depleting your body's inner resources, often without thought to the consequences. As a result, your core is weak and cold. Thus your body, in an attempt to warm itself inside, heats up erratically on the outside.*

When Kevin first explained this to me, I didn't fully understand. When he prepared an earthy herbal formula for me that completely stopped the bleeding within three days' time, I fastened onto his medicine like a lifeline. I ingested several different formulas over several years, some with similar ingredients to the first though in unique combinations. With time and fine-tuning, I no longer needed the herbs. My body continues gaining strength, and I am as active as I choose to be. I can truthfully say that, at almost sixty-one, I'm in better shape physically and mentally than I was at fifty-three when this adventure into menopause began.

During the past eight years, I have been immersed in learning to listen to my body. The shift into menopause brought with it an unsavory gain in weight, a bulk around my formerly shapely middle. With somewhat drastic dietary restrictions, I lost thirty pounds. During that time, I learned quite a bit about this miraculous physical vessel, though it took a couple of years to stabilize into a form and routine my physical self required at this point in life. All the pushing I had done in the past wasn't going to work any longer. I needed to be attentive and gentle and persistent in creating and maintaining a healthy lifestyle for my remaining years.

As a result of tuning into my body's subtle cues, I have almost completely changed my diet. While I've always prepared healthy food, baking all my own bread and cooking from scratch, I had been on automatic pilot where this body was concerned. Unknowingly, I was growing increasingly sensitive to gluten and dairy and too many fats or sweets, even those found in natural substances. In addition, I was plugging down handfuls of supplements, which experts now admit unduly tax the liver with their complexity. The body, designed to take nourishment as directly from the earth as possible, has trouble utilizing them. A preferred vegetarian, I was swilling spirulina as my main protein source, but according to the Traditional Chinese Medicine approach, this is a *cold* substance. And I needed to *warm* my interior – badly. I was drinking huge glasses of water each morning, *flooding* my kidneys, another TCM term. I was drinking water with meals, *cold* water, which was extinguishing my *digestive fire*. My body couldn't process what I was taking in, even though others might benefit from it or remain unaffected somehow. It reinforced my awareness that what is healthy for one person might actually be harmful to another.

Finally my regimen since menopause has come to include not only biweekly deep tissue massage, which I had been enjoying for several years prior, but also weekly acupuncture to help fine-tune this aging body. Trusted practitioners reinforce my inner knowing that my physical being is as sensitive as the rest of me. Between being flooded with sense impressions of violence and fear most of my early life, you could say I experience a sort of ongoing PTSD. Years later, despite various therapies, I still react to extremely slight shifts in external circumstances including the weather. My sensitivities extend as well to my own thoughts and emotions. Most surprisingly perhaps, my barometer and quirky little spiritual guide has become the dreaded hot flash. The least amount of stress that might not affect some will tip me over the edge into flushing. Knowing this, I am able to work with mindfulness, refining the practice of equanimity whenever possible. At nearly sixty-one, I experience far fewer hot flashes than I did when I began menopause at fifty-three. And I gain new awareness daily.

No matter the physical challenges (and there are many, often conflicting TCM symptoms such as *damp with dry* or *heat with cold*), I would not change a thing about aging, especially with the assistance of my wonderful healthcare partners. I have tasted true happiness, and there is no yearning to return to the angst-filled days of my youth. With age comes wisdom, if one allows it. No longer do

I frame my worth through the eyes and expectations of others. Suddenly as though I'm looking through a macro lens on a camera, what's important in life snaps sharply into focus. I don't have to dither about, floundering in indecision. My filters fall away, and I am able to confront life with clarity and directness, tempered with kindness, toward myself as well as others. And while intimacy deepens or declines with the challenges partners surely face, the opportunity ever lies in discovering another layer of unconditional love between one another. Whatever presents itself at this time in life, if it doesn't pass muster, I discover the strength to winnow it out, preparing the ground for the ultimate transition back into the vast Unknown.

What could be more exciting?

Bela Johnson

Twenty-Four

Dear you, whomever and wherever you may be,

For me the arrival of Menopause was not like this: it was *not* sudden. It was *not* what I expected. It was *not* "One day you have it, one day you don't." It was *not* a peaceful easing into the next chapter, even though that's what I'd always expected. I had thought my acceptance and "embracing" of this natural experience would make it be that way. But I was wrong. It was not like any of that. Or, I should say, it *is* not like that—present tense—because it's still evolving and I'm still living the change as it unfolds.

Before I go further, some hard facts. I'm fifty-one years old. I'm fit. I exercise every day. I fast-walk, I do yoga. I eat very well. (I live in Italy and my diet includes a lot of fresh stuff, much organic stuff and processed almost-nothing.) My weight has been the same for fifteen years. Five years ago, despite what I thought was a good foundation, things started to get wonky.

For five years things changed, felt different, weren't the way they'd been before. They call this ramping-up stage "perimenopause" which sounds sort of benign. Like a starter-marriage. Or a prolonged test-drive. Or the baby version of something more mature. And it is, sort of, all those things. Only, it's not to be discounted because it's the P-word instead of the M-word. For me, anyway, it presented its own, very real challenges. The problem was that when "its" symptoms started, I didn't know what the "it" was. I just thought that various things were wrong with me.

What things? *These* things, some of which I found very strange and scary (this is my list; yours may well be very, very different):

> The beginning of cyclical irregularity (I'd always been like a clock). Increased headaches, that started at the nape of my neck and crept around to grip the whole side of my head/jaw/ear/cheek. Intense breast tenderness, particularly on the sides (a "don't even think of touching me there" kind of tenderness). Crazy erect, super-tender nipples as if I were pregnant. Increased problems with allergies of all sorts and skin sensitivity. Bouts of dizziness, not the kind that makes you fall over, boom, but the kind that makes you feel like you just might if you're not careful. Incredible exhaustion combined with the utter inability to sleep. Or falling asleep heavily only to wake up at 2:00 or 3:00 in the morning, so wracked with a nameless anxiety that falling asleep again was impossible. Numbness in my nose, cheeks and forehead. Numbness in my lower arms and hands, particularly when sleeping. Hair falling and falling. About a year and half ago, my first experiences with hot flashes (more than one an hour). Crazy heat at night that made me rip off all covers and clothes, only to find myself freezing and naked, a half hour later. Oh, and did I mention: no sex drive whatsoever? Or the head fog? Or the feeling that half or all of my brain was stuffed with cotton for three

days at a time? Or the incredible, stupefying, comical lapses in memory?

These symptoms didn't all start at once. Nor did they last the whole five-year period. They came and went as if they'd been organized in shifts. While all this was going on my period was more or less normal, so I didn't know what it was about. I thought there was something seriously wrong with me, a cancer bouncing around indecisively, but cancers don't really do that so WTF was it? Of course, by the time the hot-flashes came I was piecing it together. But so much of it had been off-the-grid, not part of the common dialogue on the subject, I'd felt lost and confused and sort of crazy. I also felt curiously alone. Maybe it was being in a foreign country. Maybe it was not knowing how to say "Oil of Evening Primrose" in Italian for a long time, though I did figure it out. Maybe it was that my own body felt like the foreign country all of a sudden, and I was most definitely lost in translation.

A year and a half ago, I started taking natural supplements—chasteberry, pine bark extract, taurine, magnesium and melissa— which made me feel like a new (energetic, well-rested) woman. Last spring, my period stopped for 6 months, and for that 6 months I felt great. Perfect. Like the springiest of spring chickens. I thought I was in Menopause, that I had—as they say—arrived. But I was wrong.

In November, my cycle came back. The onset was worse than any PMS I'd ever had. The headaches were frequent and searing. At Christmas my body went into tilt. I got hit with a punishing sort of persistent dizziness that totally impeded my daily life. The feeling that I was going to pass out. A pressure all around my head like a tightening band. My blood pressure—forever regular and low-ish—went up and down crazily. I felt like I was going to explode. Anxiety and stress went through the roof. I felt like my internal tectonic plates weren't just shifting but crashing and crumbling. I was, despite a career of trying to maintain positivity about all things normal and natural, scared. And I felt bad.

Blood tests revealed that my hormone levels were uniformly, under-the-carpet low. I was officially, despite the vestigial menstruation, in Menopause. I'd never wanted nor expected to take hormones, but because of the dizziness and the inability to carry on with a normal, unforgiving schedule—work, children, aging parent, well, you know—I did start. And after about three weeks, I felt blessedly like myself. Almost too much. So my doctor and I lowered the dosages considerably, and I'm now down to a mere smidgeon of estrogen and progesterone. I don't want to mask either my age, nor all the symptoms I have. I want to feel where my body is, if you know what I mean. But for me, for now, that little help is necessary. My gynecologist and I will keep our eye on it, and check every now and then to see if I can go without. I'm looking forward to that. My aunt had breast cancer. I'll be checked every year. And in any case, I will not be kept on hormone replacement for more than five years.

Menopause is a process that will be in control. Not you. And this, I think, is the beauty of it. It's the right time of life to pay attention to signs and signals. To listen. To give up some fights. And to take up others.

It's strange to say after writing all of the above, but I think I might be emerging a happier, stronger person. More at peace with myself in the space-time continuum. More at peace with whatever life will throw my way. I hope.

Ciao from Milan, Italy,

Charlotte Moore

Twenty-Five

Menopause was a fairly smooth process for me but I'd like to chime in here, as anything might be useful to someone else. You never know.

My mom had a hysterectomy when I was little, and so did all my aunts. So I never had a relative to tell me about a natural experience. My mom told me she had "Hot flashes 'til I thought I'd die." But before that she was bleeding too much, for weeks at a time, and they said she was becoming anemic.

The previous years to my menopause might not have a connection, but I don't know. For me, forty-two turned out to be a pivotal year. My marriage was not a supportive and loving relationship, although it was not abusive, just two people not in love. I unintentionally fell in love with someone else online. I spent a year studying disaster preparedness, and lived out of state in a cabin for four months with three of my five kids. When I got home, I started going through Julia Cameron's *The Artist's Way*. Morning Pages were a wake-up call. I'm not exaggerating when I say that book changed my life.

The next year, my parents became very ill and died two weeks apart. The following year I got a divorce and the year after that I moved out of my ex's house and lived out of state for two years. That turned out to be rougher than I had anticipated and I moved back to be near my kids. So there were a lot of wide swings of the pendulum before things started to even out. The only reason I mention any of that is to say: pay attention. Pay attention to your moods and your relationships and your stresses. You might think you are over-reacting for no reason, but there probably is a reason. I was in a very religious home and thought it was good if I sacrificed my own interests for my family. I was homeschooling my kids and not doing anything for myself for most of those twenty-five married years. I was an artist not doing any art for a very long time. It can be very hard to find a balance, and I think working through *The Artist's Way* really helped with that. Everything was completely out of balance and it made the pendulum swings to a balanced life much more extreme.

I started noticing hot flashes when I was around 54 or so. But they weren't severe, just a bit annoying, enough to make me think, "Hmmm....I wonder."

So I did my research and started taking evening primrose oil, flaxseed oil, fish oil, Vitamin E, and got religious about all my other supplements. It's not hard to find yourself taking a handful of vitamins and supplements three times a day, especially since I was determined not to go for anything prescription.

I also found out about progesterone cream and started using that. I had to ask around how to use it, since my chiropractor didn't know. But my MD said to use it three weeks of the month and take a week off just as if I were having a regular cycle. That stopped the hot flashes. I never had them at night, and they weren't awful, but they did stop. For a couple of years I had periods six months apart. Now it's been a little over eighteen months. I stopped the progesterone cream, but I started feeling a little flashy recently so I started using it again. I get the NOW brand, it's the cheapest I've found.

I also work really hard on distinguishing between what is my business and what is not, because I learned that this is where most of my stress lies.

I would highly recommend Christiane Northrup's book, *The Wisdom of Menopause*. Maybe that is where I learned about progesterone cream. Also, *The Artist's Way*, if you feel like you're out of touch with your creative self and need to identify areas that are out of balance.

In retrospect, I think that finding my way through those other "mid-life crisis" years might have helped make my menopause easier.

Blessings to everyone as you navigate these years,

Elise K

Twenty-Six

"I don't know what to say about my menopause. I got through it pretty easy. Really don't know when I really started. Mom had some problems, she had some very heavy bleeding days. I didn't have that but I thought I would never get it over."

Grandma Farreline

Twenty-Seven

"The only thing predictable about menopause is its unpredictability." It's funny, that's what my mom told me about my periods. I had to find the humor in it so that it didn't drive me crazy. I would go months without a period and then bleed for weeks at a time. There were also times I'd get a period every two weeks then it would just disappear again. I think it started in my early 50's and lasted about five or six years. I didn't really have the hot flashes or mood swings – certainly not like Grandma did. She had such fits of rage. It was really awful. All of us kids knew what it was, but for years she insisted that she got through 'the change' without anyone ever knowing about it. Of course, we all knew – she was out of her mind mad half the time.

Fortunately I didn't experience the drastic mood swings. Initially I also thought I got away without the weight gain so many people attribute to menopause. I made it through the first few years unscathed and was feeling rather smug about it. Then one day, it was just there. Weight right around the middle that had never been there before, and it was weight that just wouldn't go away.

In the end, aside from the off and on bleeding, it really wasn't that bad. I did have a few weeks that I remember feeling sad – not because of hormones – but because that time of my life had passed. I could no longer bear children – not that I was going to have any more – but just knowing that a phase had come and gone was a little sad. I always viewed having a period, menopause and crazy hormones as the price we pay for being the sex that gets to have the pleasure of carrying around and delivering babies. It's a price I'd pay again and again. I think us ladies got the better end of that deal. Having a child is something men will never understand. We are blessed.

Marilyn

Twenty-Eight

Menopause could have cost me my life. I am a breast cancer survivor.

I am seventy-eight years old. I remember the exact time and place I had my first menopausal symptom. Hot flashes and nausea. I thought I was getting the flu. My skin was so sensitive I could only wear the thinnest cotton or linen clothes (and that in minus thirty below zero weather.) I could not bear anyone to touch me. There wasn't any real information about menopause available at that time. My gynecologist put me on hormone replacement therapy. It took more than a year to get the dosage right. During that time I was bleeding heavily and almost constantly. When the medication finally worked I was so grateful to have all the menopause symptoms end. I had no idea I would pay a terrible price because of the medication.

Seven years ago I was diagnosed with breast cancer. I was fortunate that a mammogram caught it in the very early stage. I had a lumpectomy, and six weeks of radiation. I was put on Tamoxifen. I was on Tamoxifen for three years. The side effects were so horrific I had no quality of life. I had hot flashes every twenty minutes or so – twenty-four hours a day. Every hot flash made me feel deathly ill. I refused to take Tamoxifen any longer and was put on Letrazole. The side effects of this drug were extreme joint pain. It became so debilitating I couldn't lift my arms and had problems walking. Eight months was enough so back to Tamoxifen to finish out the five years of treatment.

When I started treatment I was told I had breast cancer because of the hormone replacement therapy. I felt guilty and angry – I felt what I was going through was my fault because I wasn't strong enough to handle the symptoms of menopause. It was a bitter pill to swallow. Made doubly so because six months before I was diagnosed with breast cancer, my daughter was diagnosed with cervical cancer. All I could think was how could I look after her and deal with my cancer at the same time. I survived by focusing completely on my daughter. I nursed her, never leaving her side until she passed away at home in my arms.

So here am I. This year I will be seventy-nine years old. I am experiencing all kinds of things that no one tells you about. Menopause is part of the aging process. Time passes and other things happen to your body. Bladder control and getting up several times in the night to urinate. The lining of your vagina becomes thin – like the backs of your hands. Because of this you are prone to urinary infections. Intercourse can be painful. Taking Replens helps all this. I speak very openly to my friends and find many who didn't realize there was help for aging problems. Generally because they are too embarrassed to discuss this with their doctor or professional care giver. The internet is a wonderful source of information too. Most important I maintain a positive, cheerful attitude. I refuse to think of myself as old. Just older.

Virginia Bassett

Twenty-Nine

Am I Brave Enough? A Letter to My Sisters.

I am fifty-seven years old. And still wondering if I will ever go the promised twelve months without that wonderful menses. Both of my grandmothers are gone… or I would ask them what they experienced. My mother is physically alive but mentally and emotionally gone, so I cannot ask her either. I have no sisters, so it is me.

I am a wife, a nurse, a mother, a woman. I have just graduated with a Master's degree and am beginning a new piece of my journey ~ to teach Nursing students. This time of my life ~ when supposedly I have a part of me dying ~ taking with it hormones and chemicals that help me to function as I did in my twenties and thirties ~ this is not a sentence to stop learning, working, living, loving.

I have had some crazy moments (ask my husband), dealt with depression for a couple of years, had to have my thyroid removed in my forties, still feel like I am judged for what I look like (which is middle aged!) and not what I know or can do, and cannot believe I don't have any grandchildren yet!! But I am hopeful.

I am also an organic gardener and believe the holistic approach is the better way to go. Because of that I have not taken any hormone replacement medicine. We each have to do what is best for ourselves. I have an occasional hot flash but seem to get through it. I have noticed physical changes in my vaginal lining but it hasn't hampered anything!!! (wink, wink) All I can say is the older I get the better sex gets. (and that is all I can say!! blush, blush).

My advice, if I have any, is to do what is best for you ~ which means take the best care of yourself that you can. I know each of us gets to make our own choices and decisions but I know that my choices affect my children, my husband, my friends. Taking care of yourself means annual physical exams, monthly breast exams, walking every day, eating right and being the Woman you are meant to be at this amazing time of life. I was a hospice nurse for a few years and I had a client that taught me this valuable lesson. She was a woman in her late thirties dying from breast cancer that had metastasized to her bones and lungs. She had made the choice to do nothing when she found the lump. Nothing. I could not imagine doing nothing if I found a lump anywhere in my body. I had the hardest time understanding her choice as she had a teenage child. So please, take care of yourself.

I do not see menopause as the end but as the beginning ~ a step into a new part of my journey. This is a step for each of us to take and I wish each of you well in the journey!!!

Melinda S. Roepke

Thirty

I am fifty-seven years old and seven years down the line. I live in South Africa. My mother entered menopause about the same time as I hit puberty, I drew the short straw and was sent off to a convent boarding school. My full biology and sex education was handled by the nuns from thereon. My mother died when I was thirty, from Alzheimer's, so the subject of menopause never came up.

I married at thirty-eight and was divorced just after forty, so never had children. I had my last period just after my fiftieth and was totally relieved and liberated. I had a very busy career, stressful at times, so it was easy to blame headaches, mood swings and hot flushes on the current stress level related to work. Insomnia didn't really hassle me either, I would just get up and read or do something else.

It was at this stage that I stopped eating meat and lived mostly on raw fruit and vegetables, but my craving for bread increased dramatically. I developed psoriasis which was very difficult to control, but once I stopped work at fifty-five and readjusted my diet that has mostly cleared up. I never took any HRT or even natural therapies.

Now to find a way to get rid of this extra tummy flab that just won't move!

Laura

Thirty-One

I've seen my mom go through years of hot flashes, mood swings, all the negative aspects of menopause and then have a hysterectomy because of ovarian cancer at the age of seventy. Her difficulties lasted close to thirty-five years.

I was blessed in that I had an easy period every month and at the age of forty-eight just stopped having them. Never have had a hot flash yet and I'm now sixty-two. Never experienced mood swings or excessive anything that I saw my Mom go through. And, yes, I was terrified that I would go through the mood swings, the hatefulness, the seemingly different personalities. I cannot imagine how horrible it was for Mom to go through those things and not be able to control them. The doctors put her on a variety of medicines, vitamins, and I'm not sure what all, but they didn't seem to help. My sister and I were told that we would probably have a difficult time also. Sis did have some mood swings and hot flashes, but they were mild.

I lived with the pain of menopause through my Mom's experiences. My daughter, age forty, is going through the night sweats and hot flashes. But, I guess you could say I never really did experience menopause myself, even though technically the medical personnel say I've gone through it. I know how blessed I've been!

Katy Lamb

Thirty-Two

Dear Little Sister,

My mother did a wonderful job of informing me about what would come in puberty. Not so much with menopause however. Perhaps because menopause has so many more variations to the norm; its effects are impossible to predict. It seems no two women take the same path through The Change. And that, I think, is the first thing to understand. It is not like puberty. Its 'average ages' are much broader, and its effects are much more diverse. Only its final outcome is uniform. This is why sharing our journeys with our sisters and daughters is so very important. Hearing them may not tell us what we can expect, but hearing them helps us know we are not alone in the journey. It is a journey each of us will make if we are blessed to live long enough.

It is also important for our stories to be understood in light of the times they took place. Medical knowledge increases so quickly today that ideas and therapies from even just a decade ago are now obsolete. There is more ingenuity being brought to bear on the challenges of menopause than ever before, and for that, our daughters can be very grateful. It is not really so long ago that women were actually committed to insane asylums due to the effects of menopause. We've come a long way. So the second point I'd like to make is that you may have to assert yourself to get your concerns and needs addressed, but do it. It's your life. Keep looking for the answers you need.

My mother was born in 1935. In her mid-forties, she, like so many women in the 1970's and 80's, had a hysterectomy. With it, she crashed head-on into menopause overnight. She suffered few physical symptoms, but within days the resulting hormonal imbalance brought on a severe depression that was completely uncharacteristic for her. Although my father alerted her doctor that she was not herself, she was given no treatment. In the days that followed, her body mended but her mind did not. Five weeks later, she suddenly packed her bags and moved out. She did not even say goodbye.

It is hard to convey how utterly and completely out of character this behavior was. Mom had been happily married to her best friend for more than twenty-five years. She had a family she adored. She had work she enjoyed. And most importantly, she had a thriving, vibrant faith that was her rock solid foundation. Yet within days of her surgery, she felt unloved and empty. Foggy and adrift.

My father was heartbroken at her unexplained, unexpected rejection, but he refused to let her go without a fight. He vowed to find her and woo her back. He had captured her heart once, he would do it again. And that is what he did. After a few days, she called to let him know she was alright, and eventually she agreed to see him. They began 'dating.' Dad brought her flowers and took her for long walks on the beach. They shared malteds down at the burger joint. He called just to say good morning and good night. Slowly and gently, he won her trust. And behind the scenes, he begged her doctor to consider testing her for hormone imbalance. It took four months to convince the doctor. When he finally agreed, her numbers were 'in the cellar digging holes.' Yet it took two more months to convince Mom that she should at least try the hormone therapy.

When she finally agreed, she was herself again so quickly it felt almost instantaneous to those of us watching. The depression lifted. The fog cleared. The emptiness vanished, and Mom was back. Today, my father is eighty-six and Mom is seventy-nine. They celebrated their 62nd wedding anniversary last year. Her advice to those still new on the journey: Do not underestimate the power of hormones on your mental health.

I was twenty-five the year of Mom's surgery. I can speak with certainty about what she felt during that time because we've had many conversations about it since. Once Mom began hormone replacement therapy (HRT) and returned to her normal way of thinking, she felt guilty and somehow responsible for her depression. However in talking to other women, she's since learned just how powerful hormones are, in both our bodies and our psyche. Their influence, or lack thereof, can be completely life changing. And although I took careful notes from Mom's cautionary tale, I would feel many of the same mental effects when my turn came. Fortunately, I had learned from her experience.

Like Mom, I was told at the age of forty-three that I had a uterine fibroid. I refused the hysterectomy however and opted to have a myomectomy instead, removing just the fibroid and leaving all my plumbing intact. It was an option I had to fight for, because my gynecologist insisted hysterectomies are so much "easier." He never mentioned the fact that many women experience intercourse very differently without their uterus. And for some, the uterus is even an integral part of a satisfying sex life. So I guess the question is, "easier" for whom? Personally, I'm glad I didn't cave in to his pressure.

It was immediately after my surgery that doctors found I shared another similarity to my Mom. Although I'd never had hypertension previously, I needed a prescription to control it even before I left the hospital. And my blood pressure has never normalized to this day. When I did a little research, I found that this is a not-so-uncommon side effect of uterine surgery of any kind. My sister would later experience the same exact thing. It can be immediate, like ours, or appear gradually over a couple of months, but I would caution you to check your blood pressure regularly if you do have any uterine surgery.

For me, The Change began some time in my early forties. By forty-four, I had hot flashes that woke me from a dead sleep multiple times during the night. Of course, I had them during the day too, but the night time ones woke me so fully, and happened so repeatedly, that I suffered from chronic sleep deprivation. At the time however, I was unaware of just how exhausted I'd become. It's only after you return to normal that you realize how tired you really were.

Yet the most impactful effect I experienced from

menopause was one I never associated with The Change. Early in my forties I had begun "ummming." I would look at my husband or my kids, meaning to tell them something and then, as quickly as the thought had come, it was gone. While they looked at me expectantly, all I could do was whisper "uuummmm," as I furrowed my brow and furiously tried to recapture the elusive thought. Sometimes, I could retrieve it. Often I could not. This got to be such a regular occurrence that it became a kindly joke. My kids, both teenagers, would say, "Mom, you're ummming." And I would answer, "Yes I know, it will come to me." But frequently it did not.

In fact, from 'ummming,' I moved to serious forgetfulness. I completely forgot important errands and appointments. Reading a novel became impossible. I couldn't even watch a movie because I couldn't remember the plot. A heavy fog engulfed my brain. I couldn't carry on a normal conversation at times, because I couldn't follow the train of thought. I could not stay focused, and found myself rudely interrupting people in order to speak before I forgot what I wanted to say. I also found it very difficult to filter my thoughts from my speech, so I often said things as they popped into my mind. Unfortunately this was especially true when I was nervous or stressed. I was honestly beginning to fear that I was experiencing the first stages of early-onset Alzheimer's. It never once occurred to me that my symptoms might be related to menopause.

By forty-six, however, the hot flashes drove me to my gynecologist. They had become quite debilitating, and I had tried a number of herbal remedies and vitamin regimens with no success at all. The doctor did a blood test and confirmed that I was completely menopausal. I had not had a period in over a year, and all my hormone levels were in the fully menopausal range. When I asked what he recommended, he replied, "Be patient. It will pass eventually." I truly wanted to crawl over his desk and strangle him with his own ridiculous Donald Duck tie.

Fortunately, that same day I also had an appointment with my regular M.D. After the usual routine, he asked if I had any other concerns. I explained about the hot flashes and exhaustion, and my previous appointment with my gynecologist. I asked if he knew anything that might help. When he recommended hormone replacement therapy, I wanted to kiss his feet. Yes, there are increased risks associated with HRT. And yes, it is not a decision to make lightly. However, I was so very grateful for the option.

For me, the effects of HRT were nothing short of miraculous. The hot flashes stopped completely and I was sleeping through the night again within three days. But the unexpected benefit was even better: I could think again! I could remember! The 'ummmming' stopped!! My family noticed immediately. I no longer had trouble following a conversation, or a movie plot. I could read a book! I could even remember more complex things that I realized I hadn't been able to do since my late thirties. The difference has been absolutely life-altering. Today I am fifty-eight, and the fog and memory issues have not returned. I am still on HRT, although not at the same doses, and my doctor monitors me carefully.

On a side note, my doctor shared with me that until my case, he was unaware of just how drastic menopausal memory loss can be. Now he asks patients about it specifically and finds it's more common than he expected, although not usually as severe as mine. Yet, like me, many women don't initially associate memory loss and 'fogginess' with hormone imbalance. Instead, they believe it's just a natural part of getting older. Of course, not all memory issues are connected to menopause, but sometimes they are.

Finally, I do not share my story as an endorsement of HRT. It is not for everyone. Despite the risks however, it is the best choice for some of us. Rather, I want to endorse not giving up. Not letting some guy in a white coat tell you to "Be patient. This will pass eventually." It's your life. Network. Talk to friends, and mothers of friends if possible. Latch onto that woman nodding knowingly as you fan yourself on the bus. You'll be surprised what you can learn from a total stranger. Talk to family. If you can't talk to your mother, try another family member. Even cousins may know something about family tendencies you do not. Information is power. Don't be afraid to ask 'dumb' questions. Go online. Talk to your medical professionals. Educate yourself. Listen to your body. Keep searching.

Barb

Thirty-Three

I took the natural way through it all, and had no one to give me advice (yep, I also have a mother who preferred not to talk about 'those kind of things' — heck she doesn't even like it when someone says *breast!!*). Luckily enough the great Internet was just starting up and I could do research on my own. Took me awhile and a lot of experiments, but I came up with a herbal solution that fit my needs.

Mainly things like black cohash, fenugreek, B vitamins, evening primrose oil, etc. I certainly don't miss my reproduction years — had two children before the age of twenty-three, and that was fine with me. Suffered badly with the monthly periods, with a good dose of migraines, cramps, bloating, the whole nine yards! Now I may get the odd hot flush, which is wonderful in the winter (especially winters like we just had) and maybe night sweats, but that may be just because I don't have air conditioning, and it can get pretty darn hot during the summer nights.

But these are hardly things I worry about. Luckily I have always been a very open minded person and do not find any subject taboo, so my daughter has all the information and knows she only has to ask if she needs more.

Just a side note — do you know why they call it *hysterectomy?* Because back in the day the so called medical geniuses found that a woman going through menopause was often prone to hysterics, so they reasoned that if you removed all the 'womanly' bits it would cure her! Either that or she ended up in a nut house!! Not kidding, many a woman who ended up in a mental institution was sent there because she was having a hard time with menopause and the men in her life (husband and doctor) thought she had completely lost it.

Lyn

Thirty-Four

I remember my mom going through menopause.

I want to say she was in her mid-forties. The skies darkened, thunder clapped, lightening flashed, fire and brimstone rained upon our earth and burnt our crops. Don't get me wrong, there were some bad days, too.

It was around the time we got our first computer with Internet.

We were all obsessed with chat rooms: the idea of connecting with people on the other side of the world and anywhere in between was thrilling. We all chatted in the same public room as we took turns on the computer. My mom had become friends with a couple in another state. Because we had to share our one computer, they started talking on the telephone. She became very sullen, which wasn't like her. She started taking St. John's Wort as an herbal remedy for depression, which was also unlike her.

One day she got an email from the wife telling her to stop contacting them because it was causing problems with their own relationship. She cried for a month straight! I had never seen my mother cry unless there was a dire crisis over which she had no control, certainly not over a silly failed friendship! One day just before Christmas she blurted through her tears "I just want you to know that I love Bill very much and would never leave him or break up our family." What?! Where the heck did that come from?

I was in my mid-twenties, and Bill was just my step-dad, so my family had been long broken. What in the world are you talking about, woman?! She stayed depressed, despite her St. John's Wort, for four months. I didn't see her cry ever again but she was sad and mopey that whole time. So very, very unlike her and I wished so much that I could have slapped some sense into her. I know that during this time she was bleeding whole oceans. The bleeding stopped when the depression did.

Just like that it seemed to stop.

Janine Ann

Thirty-Five

I battled with severe endometriosis from the time I started menstruation. After more than a decade of laparoscopic surgeries, numerous drug therapies, and horribly painful periods I finally had a hysterectomy at thirty years old, but kept my ovaries. I assumed menopause would be the normal process of the ovaries shutting down and the adrenal glands taking over as the major source of hormone production. For this reason I was unwilling to seek hormone replacement therapy. This seemed to be the course of nature, so why interfere with that?

At the age of forty-six, I began experiencing night sweats. That lasted for two years. And really, the night sweats were the worst of menopause symptoms for me. No wonder insomnia is common with menopause – who can sleep drenched in sweat every night? There were other bothersome symptoms like fatigue, and occasional hot flashes sometimes accompanied by waves of nausea. I was more emotional than usual. I spent a lot of time weeping or getting fired up about something or over nothing. More alarming was a fluctuating libido, vaginal dryness, and urinary incontinence (frequency and stress).

Then there were issues that I wasn't sure accompanied menopause or if I was just showing signs of age. My memory slipped more and my thought process seemed slower. Sometimes my mind seemed to just go blank! I wondered if I had early-onset Alzheimer's. My already dry skin was requiring heavier moisturizers, and seemed to be less elastic overall. Wrinkles appeared and so had these tiny little age spots. Suddenly my vision took a dive and I had to get reading glasses! It was like overnight, someone flipped a switch, and everything changed!

Menopause prompted me to look at life differently. I was not willing to accept that what I was experiencing had to continue in misery or had to be negative. I did not want to use the excuse that I was going through 'The Change' when one of my symptoms popped up. I was not willing to rely solely on information from my doctor or even friends. Instead, I was prompted to investigate how I could make the best of what my body was going through and do it naturally. I could rebel against this and be miserable or I could discover how to roll with it.

I have made changes in my lifestyle that have improved or abolished every one of the symptoms. I follow a healthy diet (my husband and I follow the Paleo lifestyle). I indulge in a nap when I need one. I keep active outdoors with gardening and yard work and I spend plenty of time enjoying nature. Simple Kegel exercises stopped the incontinence issue. I learned to dress in layers and keep from conditions or foods that prompted hot flashes. I decided to laugh at my forgetfulness and keep notepads handy to jot down thoughts or lists I might need later. For me, the biggest difficulty was getting my stress levels under control. Better coping skills have helped me to deal with daily frustrations, and avoid the triggers. I simplified my life so that the daily load wasn't so heavy. I'm convinced the moodiness associated with menopause is just plain overload of a stressful life.

I also found it very beneficial to have someone to talk to. A compassionate and loving spouse, relative or friend goes a long way on the days when you just feel crazy.

Menopause has been a wakeup call for me. It isn't just something that 'happens' to us. It's not a disease or a label or a problem. It is a shift or progression to another phase in life. Menopause is part of the aging process I accept and embrace. What you create is how the experience will be for you.

My fifties have been my best years yet.

It is all about perspective!

Love from southwest Oklahoma,

Lori Lynn

Thirty-Six

We lived in Kansas City during the 1970's, when Mom went through menopause. It was a metropolitan area with plenty of doctors and hospitals and modern technology. I can find no excuse for my mom's doctor.

Mom was raised on a farm in rural Michigan during the depression. She worked hard as a child and put herself through a couple years of college. She raised my oldest brother on her own during a time when that was not so common and worked as a bookkeeper for the local paper.

After she married my dad, she became a stay-at-home mom. I'm not sure she ever sat down except to watch her stories during lunch. She cooked three meals a day for us and the house was so clean I had trouble getting my housekeeping badge in Girl Scouts. She taught piano, was active in the church, and was an artist. When she broke her leg, she bounced up and down the stairs on her bottom to do laundry instead of waiting for one of us to help. She was a breast cancer survivor. What I'm trying to say is that she was a strong woman.

When menopause hit, Mom wasn't about to sit down and feel sorry for herself. It was not an easy time for her. She essentially hemorrhaged for more than two years. There wasn't a lot of cycle to it she just bled constantly. She wouldn't stop doing the things she had to do, so when she felt a clot coming, she grabbed a plastic bag to catch it. She had mood swings and who could blame her? I sometimes found her in the basement crying. Not very often, she was too tough to let that show.

She did not go to the doctor often; it took something pretty awful to get her to go. She was weak and exhausted and, I think, anemic. And her doctor told her the constant bleeding and the large clots were normal and to stop complaining. I'm not sure I can ever really forgive him for that. I don't know exactly what he said but it came across as- stop being such a girl.

I can't remember how long it took but she did not give up. She eventually saw a gynecologist who told her that what she was experiencing was NOT normal. He was appalled. She had two D&Cs and it was over.

I've wondered whether the aggressive breast cancer treatment Mom had in the 70's somehow made menopause worse for her. But I have a friend who had much the same experience. She told me that she would lay in the shower for hours, letting the clots pass.

So I dreaded menopause (or perimenopause). Not that I'm not totally ready to be done with the whole monthly bleeding thing, but the only women I knew who had talked about it were my mom and that one friend and they both had such a difficult experience. My experience ended up being on the other end of the spectrum, really rather boring. I like to think of it as normal. Normal is usually pretty boring.

I think people are much more likely to tell the horror

stories, like Mom's, rather than the boring stories like my own. Mom's story is far more interesting, but here goes. I started skipping periods a few years ago. Sometimes I had a really heavy period, when I did have one, and that was a little frustrating. For the previous ten years or so, my periods had decreased to 1-2 days per month of really light bleeding. So when I started having 5-6 days of heavy bleeding every few months, I whined. But the time between started stretching further and further apart and the periods I did have were much lighter and only lasted a couple days.

I really don't have much to complain about, I just wish it was over. I went a full year without a period and just when I thought I was done my body surprised me. Now I have another full year to wait to be officially in menopause. One month down.

Eleven to go.

Nancy Anderson

Thirty-Seven

My name is Marie. I am a sixty-seven year old Irish woman living in County Antrim for the past thirty-seven years (top right hand corner of the map of Ireland, but actually part of the UK). I was born and reared about a hundred miles further south, in Dublin, the capital of the Republic of Ireland.

I grew up in a rather typical Irish Catholic family – six children, my mother had nine pregnancies in total, two miscarriages and a baby that survived for only five hours. Mammy never carried any of us for more than seven months. So, if you like, we were not exactly textbook babies, your normal 'nine-monthers!'

I certainly did not have a textbook body and coming from Holy Catholic Ireland- sure it was almost sinful to make any mention of periods, menstruation, the menstrual cycle, or 'the curse.' As for heavy periods, painful periods, irregular periods, periods that stop and abnormal bleeding between periods…those would call for extra penance if mentioned in confession. There were, of course, hushed whispered conversations between the older women in the family, but we children were not meant to hear them.

As you know a half story is more dangerous than the full story! Particularly when it comes to 'Wimmins stuff!'

Any books I read told me that:

> *Periods usually start to occur around the same time as other changes happen to the body, such as starting to*

develop breasts or to grow pubic hair. The average age to start periods is 13, but it is normal to start at any time between the ages of 11 and 15. Periods continue until the menopause, which is usually around the age of 50 years.

Well, there you go, I was NOT normal! I was one of the late starters. A very late starter. Twenty-one years of age and still with a chest like a pastry board, bald as a coot down below and muscles like sparrow's kneecaps – a skeleton with skin on. A pretty picture. Not!

My periods were very heavy, irregular and double-up painful from the word go. The solution? Physical work and just keep going. Sympathy? Not at all, sure we did not talk about it and nobody else could feel my pain. Is it any wonder that at age thirty one, when my daughter was born, I proclaimed childbirth was easier than the pain I put up with every month!

Mammy had an easy time with menstruation, a bleed for three or four days from the age of sixteen. At the age of forty-one after my sister was born, her periods never returned. No symptoms, life just continued. Two years after my sister was born, Mammy had a heart attack – a problem that troubled her for the rest of her life, although she managed to stick around until, at eighty-two years of age, she had a stroke and died ten weeks later.

Three years after my daughter was born, the word and symptoms of menopause raised their ugly head. I went to see my local doctor armed with a list as long as a month of Sundays.

Hot flushes/flashes.
Night sweats greater than a tsunami every hour of the night.
Vaginal dryness.
Loss of libido.
Mood swings.
Tears at the drop of a hat.
Skin like sandpaper.
Hair like straw.
Nausea.
No appetite.
No taste.
Feeling exhausted.
Unable to sleep.
Being clumsy.
Letting dishes fall.
Burning food.
Lack of concentration.
Snapping at my darling patient husband.
Shouting at my daughter.

Did he help?

Not one tiny bit. The doctor said that I was too young for the menopause and to come back in a couple of years if the symptoms persisted! Dinner preparation was a noisy affair that day and fortunately there was nobody about to hear me. I banged the pots on to the cooker (I think I have a chip in the enamel to this very day), I shouted at the walls, peeled spuds through my tears but was calmed down by the time my husband arrived to enfold me in his arms and give me comfort and wipe away my fresh round of tears.

I persevered. I waited a year before going back to the doctor, but when I saw him I was prepared to sit in his office all day, until he did some tests. It was in the days before we had Internet search engines, and the library in the small town where I lived had little in the way of self-help books.

At that consultation he told me he had been reading up on the subject of menopause.

"There is some new thinking, statistics showed that women who were late starters, like you, were often early finishers!" he had said, adding, "The good news is that women who had a difficult menopause, were less likely to have a heart attack."

I was at a later stage, to prove him wrong on both counts. I discovered that my father's eldest sister was a late starter like me (at age twenty-one) and her periods lasted until she was sixty. The neck of my womb was way over and just south of my Right hip bone. And I had a mild stroke a week after my daughter's wedding.

All the 'natural health' remedies he suggested, I had tried without any improvement. So he took me down the HRT route. It did help. Notice I said 'help' and not cure. It reduced rather than removed all the symptoms. My husband could sleep in a dry bed again without the tsunami waves drowning him. A very young Elly even noticed the difference. One morning when she saw me taking my medication, she asked, "Mammy, are these tablets to make you happy again?" She was FIVE! My husband was happy and my daughter was happy to have 'mammy' back.

I, on the other hand, though pleased with the improvement, noticed that when the 'rest stage' from the pills happened, the symptoms returned with a vengeance. It was as if the pills suppressed and kept them on hold. Still, a week of symptoms was far better than all day every day.

At one stage, the doctor suggested me taking the HRT for three straight months without a break, stop for one week and repeat. Life got better, but the break weeks were a tsunami of symptoms that hit with a mighty surge.

I soldiered on for many years. In my mid forties, my husband was diagnosed with terminal cancer, and he became my sole 24/7 career. I lost sleep, energy, and weight. My periods stopped and I gave a great big sigh of relief. I spoke to the doctor and he agreed that I should stop the HRT. My husband died when I was fifty one and two months later the periods restarted with most of the aforementioned symptoms. After a year they became more erratic but only finished when I was fifty-eight.

Painkillers never eased my 'doubled-up' pain. I found a hot water bottle at my tummy and a teaspoon full of brandy did the trick. A towel over my body, tucked under my arms and between my legs soaked up the sweat.

Grannymar

Thirty-Eight

Menopause was easy for me. The only tip I got from a doctor or nurse practitioner was that estrogen is stored in fat so menopause can be easier on women who weigh a little more than the very thin women our culture admires. She said if I weighed ten pounds extra I would have an easier time. She was right.

I didn't actually have to gain weight because I tend to be a little plump. I had a few night sweats, often brought on by eating chocolate or drinking coffee, but I never had a hot flash, mood swings, or any of the other things they like to terrify you with. I don't miss washing out my underwear or having to change the sheets all of the time or having to shell out money for supplies.

I was a little worried that sex would feel odd after menopause, but when I got around to meeting Johnny everything was fine. My sum total of experience: no big deal, nothing to worry about (but it is not the same for other women necessarily – my thin Mom had it rough). I also never took artificial hormones (birth control pills), which may have helped – not taking them, I mean.

Sharyn Dimmick

Thirty-Nine

My mother was forty-five the year I was born (the youngest of eight children), and my three older sisters are eighteen, fifteen and eight years older than me. So no information from my mother or my sisters – menopause was not something that was talked about.

I had a hysterectomy at forty-one because of major endometriosis, but my gynecologist left my ovaries so I wouldn't be thrown into immediate menopause. She is the one who answered my questions about menopause (bless her). She did say that generally menopause would start around age fifty.

I have had a few hot flashes. I don't sleep well, but that is the extent of it. I have learned that my personal consumption of sugar, caffeine and processed foods make the symptoms worse. So I follow a Paleo meal plan for the most part.

Jean

Forty

Dearest Little Sister of Cecilia,

I wish to open this letter to you by saying what a remarkable and wonderful sister you have. Cecilia is loved by so many in the blogosphere; she has brought the good, bad and sad of farming and being self sufficient to so many of us who would ordinarily have been none the wiser and each of her daily posts is like sitting in the kitchen with Cecilia, enjoying a cuppa, while she tells us about her day.

My name is Mandy Frielinghaus, and I live in the Eastern Cape of South Africa in a little village called Cannonville, Sundays River. I am in my early forties and have a loving husband who sadly has to travel far too much for business. Our three cats who are my children keep me company while Pete is away.

I have wonky hormones from having a bicornuateunicollis uterus – all that really means is I don't have one uterus, I have two. Just like all other woman, I only have one cervix and one set of fallopian tubes with the difference of two independent uteruses. Even due to my 'condition,' I have a regular 28-day cycle, despite not being on any form of contraception. My husband had a vasectomy when he was twenty-seven (which was before I met him), after having two children, so naturally there has never been a need for me to take pregnancy preventative measures. Sadly I don't have any children but that is a story for another day and one I share in my book, well, that is if I ever get it finished.

From my late teens through mid twenties, I had laparoscopic surgeries done to firstly ascertain the condition of my uteruses and whether it was best to remove one or both – turns out both were perfectly fine. Over a number of years, I had a few surgeries done to remove fibroids and bilateral tumors on my ovaries (the size of oranges) which mostly consisted of bone hair and teeth! I know, it sounds terrible. Due to my oddball hormones, my chromosomes got a bit confused and formed what they thought was a pregnancy in my ovaries. Thankfully all seems to have settled and here I am now in the throes of perimenopause with sensitive tender breasts, bloating, nausea, fatigue, loss of libido, trouble sleeping through the night, sore joints, headaches, forgetfulness, some hot flushes, being somewhat moody every now and again and crying for silly reasons – on the upside though, my period is a lot lighter. This all sounds very bleak but it is amazing what a positive attitude can do. Not for one minute am I saying any of this is always a walk in the park but I am definitely of the belief that your outlook can make or break any situation.

My mom went through menopause when she was fifty and she says it was a doddle with nothing more than irregular periods; spotting here and there and the occasional what she would not even class as a hot flush. I hope that both you and I can experience menopause just as my mom did, as I know there are woman who suffer through so much until they are on the other side of it all.

With love from a sunny South Africa,

Mandy Frielinghaus

Forty-One

I'm writing at my kitchen table in a tiny village in Eastern Ontario. It's pouring rain and warming up slowly after the longest, snowiest winter in many a year. I am now in my sixty-fifth year so menopause, except for the occasional mild hot flash, is behind me. Menopause happened in two stages in my case because my womb was removed when I was forty-two – but not my ovaries (thankfully).

The end of bleeding came as a great relief after a truly awful menstrual history. There were a couple of surprises, though. One was that it was years before I learned to stop dreading the surprise onset of always heavy periods. The more profound surprise was the intensity of my grief at the ending of my life as a fertile woman, even though I had two children and my husband had had a vasectomy some years before.

As my ovaries continued to function, the rest of the menopause story didn't begin to unfold for another eight years.

I had asked my mother about her Change. She said she didn't even realize what was happening she had so few symptoms. I don't think she was being coy with me. In fact, I remember her saying that she was terrified that she was pregnant with a sixth child when her periods stopped.

So I only knew what I'd read, which wasn't much. Looking back, I think I didn't have too bad a time of it.

Being hot all the time was bizarre as, up until then, my tendency was to be on the chilly side. And the term 'hot flash' doesn't even begin to describe the experience! I'd never experienced wringing wet slimy palms before – yuck!

A significant increase in libido was pretty disconcerting, especially as my husband found it off-putting. This has tapered off over time but as someone else remarked, even though mentally I'm not much interested, the body still likes it occasionally.

The hardest things for me to deal with were the night sweats and disruption to sleep and the weight gain. However I did have the attitude that all fell within the range of normal changes and Mother Nature has her reasons.

I think that the old term The Change is apt. Everything is different after the drama. We begin to take on our final role, that of the 'elder woman' - this term was coined by Marian Van Eyck Maccain. It doesn't have the baggage that 'crone' carries.

Susan

Forty-Two

A Journey of Change

My journey begins with a hysterectomy at age thirty-three. I was diagnosed with cervical cancer and given the option by a gynecological oncologist to undergo ridiculously horrible sounding radiation treatments whereby some device emitting who knows how much radiation would be discretely inserted into my vagina to blast away the cancer cells.

"No thank you," I said. "I have children. I don't plan to have anymore. Get rid of my uterus and if need be, my ovaries as well."

Saying goodbye to those female parts was obviously not an issue for me. At least it was much less of an issue than the alternative.

Fortunately, my ovaries were clean and so my real road down the menopause path was partially averted. I got to keep producing lady hormones with all the advantages of never having a menstrual period again.

It is important to note, mainly because no one ever told me this and someone has to say it that after your uterus is removed, orgasms are never quite the same. An orgasm with a uterus is profound, deep, overwhelming. An orgasm without a uterus is just okay, nothing to brag about.

Since half the work of menopause was artificially accomplished for me I think I was relatively lucky. Have you heard the word peri-menopause? If not, it just means the warm up period before the real event. Some women experience bits and pieces and symptoms years before they actually step down the road to the finish line. Not having a period often provided entertainment and mystery as I would guess and wonder and reflect on symptoms that maybe, might be, no-not really, but could be- the beginning of the end.

Little things really: some changes in bathroom habits, some weight gain, some skin changes, some hot flashes (more on this coming), and most significantly and most welcome: the end of hormone induced migraine headaches!

This all began at about forty-eight years of age. Within a few years more weight crept onto my 5'6" frame. My skin became thinner, drier, and dark brown blotches were creating roadmaps for me to trace designs over and under and around body parts. My hair got thinner, then it slowed in growth, then I didn't have to shave anymore, then my pubic hair began to thin. No one ever told me about this either. Standing in front of a mirror I reasonably resemble a slightly overweight, saggy skinned, pubic hair challenged ten year old girl with graying hair—and yes, the hair that is left "down there" is turning gray as well.

Finally, back to those hot flashes I mentioned. What I experienced in peri-menopause were not hot flashes. Menopausal hot flashes roll over your body from the inside out. Literally. I want you to imagine being set on fire from within your chest. Now feel those flames spreading up your neck, around to your back, and out your extremities. Of course nothing is visible, but you are on fire and cooking from the inside out. Then the sweat comes: soaking, dripping, drenching sweat. These episodes happen a lot at 3am. They also happen in the middle of the day, at your place of work, while you are driving. You have no control. That is the hard part. You can't plan them you can't stop them. You just have to roll with them.

I am now fifty-four and I am finished. My journey is over.

The exciting news for you- not every women experiences symptoms. That's the great thing. We are all unique and wonderful in our bodies. The other great thing- we are women and we cope. We persevere. We work with what our bodies give to us and we triumph.

We reflect on our lives, our happiness and sorrow, our dreams and desires. We grow within ourselves and grow our minds. We create. We change yes, but it is up to each one of us to decide how we change and what path our journey will take.

Where will your journey take you? I wish you the best as you travel.

All the best from Washington,

Debbie Tecca

Forty-Three

This past December was one year since I had my last period. My periods were horrific for the last ten years because I had fibroids and the only option offered to me was a hysterectomy, which I refused after doing a lot of research. Would you believe one doctor told me they would turn cancerous? That's a flat out lie. I also found out that recent studies show women who have had hysterectomies have shorter lives by five to ten years. Even after menopause, those reproductive organs serve a purpose. There are better treatments for fibroids now, but they were not yet thought of or were experimental during the time period when I could have used them.

My mother had a hysterectomy when she was in her forties. It was the done thing in those days. After having five children, the doctor told her she'd be better off yanking everything out. That way, he said, she wouldn't have to worry about ovarian or uterine cancer as she aged. I never got the time or chance to ask her if she experienced any kind of menopausal symptoms. By the time I was starting to go through it, Mom was diagnosed with lung cancer. I guess she could have kept her uterus and ovaries after all (although, after having five children and adhering to Catholic principles, it was probably a relief to her not to have to deal with the possibility of pregnancy again). My mother died in 2009, three years before I officially became menopausal, and the one time I did ask her about it, she shooed away the question and said she hadn't experienced any problems at all.

I've had hot flashes on and off for over ten years, but in December of 2012, after my last bleeding time, the hot flashes turned nuclear. I am positive that one day I will spontaneously combust. My husband will come home from work one day and find nothing remaining of me except soot on the ceiling and ashes on the floor. For a few weeks last year, the hot flashes were accompanied by waves of extreme anxiety. I worked hard not to resort to pharmaceuticals. I know too much about them from being married to a pharmacologist and from my years working in a pharmacy. (That said, I know that sometimes we all need a little help, and if I had to, if all else failed, I would get a prescription for something that would assist me through the worst of the anxiety. I also know that for some, medication is a godsend so I most certainly don't judge or begrudge the use of drugs when necessary.) I got up early and established a morning routine of yoga, meditation, exercise (cardio to get those endorphins flowing), walks outside, reading (to learn, to be inspired, to distract myself from myself), and writing in my journal. I ate healthful, nourishing, nurturing foods. For me, that meant being mostly vegetarian. I do eat some soy, but only the fermented varieties (tofu, tempeh, miso). It worked. Then I failed to maintain it these past few months so I'm back to having some anxiety with my hot flashes. That means I need to get back on track.

Insomnia has become almost constant, partially because of the hot flashes. They are at their worst at night. Between 1:00 and 4:00 AM, I hot flash and can't sleep. I have stopped worrying about it. Every third night or so, I'll be exhausted enough to sleep well. I consider it a blessing.

I recently had the opportunity to spend a weekend with some older female friends who were wonderfully supportive, and able to give me advice on what I'm experiencing. Better yet, they reassured me that this is normal.

Just hearing that was comforting.

Robin Simmons

Forty-Four

My mom went through menopause at age thirty-nine, and even though she is still with me (now eighty-six) she was unable to share anything about her experience other than her age when she went through it. She simply said it was no big deal for her, no issues that she could remember. She did say that she was told that women who had children went through it earlier that those that did not. I have no sisters to compare notes with or other older female relatives to consult, so I have no additional familial history for a basis of comparison, but here is my experience.

Multiple doctors told me over the years that as a daughter, I will probably go through menopause at about the same age that my mother did, but this wasn't true for me. I will be fifty-four later this year, have no children and menopause began for me around age fifty-one.

In the beginning, I had a few night sweats and some noticeable hormone surges and mood swings… to which my husband could attest. I also experienced some forgetfulness. I was far more prone to weepiness during this time and I would get unusually flushed in the face sometimes, for no apparent reason, but it would subside fairly quickly. And, unlike most side effects I've read, I had some minor adult onset acne (I did not have any as a teen), which my dermatologist said was normal with the hormone changes. I've also noticed less elasticity and more dryness of my skin, which may just be a symptom of age. But all in all, nothing terribly debilitating, just noticeable. The worst thing for me during this time and ongoing, has been some progressive weight gain and "rearranging" around the middle, which I'm still fighting and it doesn't want to leave!

I've had fibroids for many years, which impact your periods even when you are on the pill, and I was told that they would shrink at menopause. Perhaps they have, I can't really say at this point. The tapering off of my periods, which were quite heavy during this time, was very disconcerting. First, I didn't have one for six months, then I'd have one every other month for the next four months, and then go many months again without one, and then surprise! This went on for about a year and a half. At this point, I haven't had a period for seventeen months and was told that if you go eighteen months you're officially "through" menopause, though many doctors say this is true after twelve months. I have never taken any hormones for menopausal symptoms, just regular vitamins.

On the up side of this time of life, I can say that I'm experiencing a renewed sense of empowerment, confidence and some found energy that is really exciting. In some ways I feel younger now than I did in my forties, and certainly view things more clearly than ever before. It really feels like there is another dimension of the world and of life to experience and explore. Perhaps this is somewhat age related, but I feel kind of liberated now that I don't worry about my periods, and I want to embrace and enjoy this phase of my life.

Betsy

Forty-Five

Late Thoughts on Menopause

For me menopause (what is the verb—"arrived," "visited," "swept in"?) in 2002, so when I decided to write this piece, I thought I had some perspective on and distance from it. I thought, menopause was not dramatic; I did not melt down or fall apart or feel anguish or even spend a lot of time thinking about it. But, not trusting to memory, I dug out one of my journals from that year to see what I was writing about. I was surprised to learn that I'd "forgotten" so much of that time. I read that I was angry in my marriage, dissatisfied with my work, worried about my sons, and frustrated with my lack of time and space to do what really mattered to me. I felt shackled. I wanted change in my life. I wanted to change myself. No wonder the popular euphemism for menopause is "the change of life."

Five things helped me illuminate this time in my life and even to appreciate it: reading, writing, dreaming, meditating, and talking to my sister and friends who were "going through" (as in a phase, as in a passage) menopause. These five things were interactive and if there was a shape to things it was a spiral—that is, we would talk with each other about our reading, writing, dreaming, and meditating, which helped us go deeper in our understanding, which in turn informed our writing and dreams. Each insight went into the spiral, things circled around but at another level. I began to see menopause not as a single turning point but as a series of moments that accumulated, offering insights along the way. I wanted to consciously move through it, and I find that its particles of wisdom continue to trail me, and perhaps will for the rest of my life.

My "sister" conversations would cover everything from the superficial to the profound: *Are you going to color (or to continue to color) your hair as it goes gray? Is your skin dry? Are you finding your life dull? Are you tired of feeling stressed? I am angry. I cry for no reason. Sometimes I hate my husband. Is this dress too young for me? How is your sex life? Am I too old to flirt without looking ridiculous? I found a great product, all natural. I found a great book. You need to see this movie. My sister told me. I am leaving my job. I am going to Tibet. I don't care about all that anymore.*

In addition to my close friends, I was also part of a moon circle—a monthly gathering of women who shared what was going on in our lives. We talked about our lives, our dreams, archetypes, wondered how to transition sanely from mother to crone (yet resisting "crone," a word that made us feel old and ugly). We would not let history or the media define or diminish what we were experiencing. We had outgrown youth, with its coquetry and desirability, constantly being marketed to or our images sold as commodities. As feminists we scorned all that, but some of it still clung to us like cobwebs. We do not want to *look old*. What was it we were becoming? Not "matrons" or "spinsters." "Wise women" was better. "Witches" had power and mystery. Names were important; we needed the right words to help us claim being women of a certain experience and knowledge. This was an initiation.

And there was wisdom that went beyond words. In addition to our talks, we performed a ritual each month, often raising our voices in collective, spontaneous singing. These songs without words came from places deep in each of our bodies. As they braided together they became more than the sum of our parts. They were incantations, and it felt as if we had tapped into an ancient female consciousness.

I wrote in my journal about a Latin American vocalist I saw performing with a trio, who was probably in her sixties: *She wore dangling earrings, jangly bracelets, a low-cut blouse, and deep red lipstick. She sang with passion, experience, subtlety, sexuality, confidence, and ease. She and her art were one. That is how I'd like to be at her age. To know my own power, be comfortable with it. Speak, sing, honestly, live my values. Claim my self.*

I think of menopause as "unbecoming." In this I reclaim the word: I mean it not in the sense of being unattractive, but in letting go of (much of) what we spent most of our lives in becoming—that is, what others expected us to be.

Just as the beginning of menstruation jump-started me into realizing I was in unchartered territory, a scary yet exciting landscape ("today you are a woman"—yikes!), so did the end of it. Only rather than looking ahead, wondering what kind of life awaited me, I found myself looking back, wondering what kind of life I have had so far. During this menopausal year I did consciously *pause*. One son was living on his own, the other was about to graduate from high school. My role as a mother was changing, and had been changing for the last few years. My marriage was changing. I was changing. My work life was frenzied, filled with responsibility and stress, yet I did not feel valued. The world after 9/11 felt confusing, tumultuous, scary, reactive. In various ways I was asking, Is the way I am living my life what I really want? If not, do I have the courage to transform it? Myself? As Tracy Chapman sang, "If not now, when?"

To say, "When I reached menopause …" has a physicality, as in reaching a destination. I think of a mesa—a high, flat place with an amazing vista. I looked down at my life and saw myself at different ages; I could see where I'd come from and, possibly, where I might be going.

And where I was at that time. I wanted to break out of certain behavioral patterns. I wanted to live a more authentic life, which meant speaking the truth, which meant being less fearful, more creative, doing things that invited joy.

I continued my daily walking and yoga practice and began a meditation practice. In yoga I was reminded that I am not my mind or my body, but that my body is a dwelling place for the spirit within. Through yoga I experienced peace and took time to feel gratitude. I realized that most of my life I had been striving for self-improvement. When I asked my meditation teacher how to align this striving with the Buddhist concept of No Self, he suggested that I start with the thought that I am OK just as I am. What? Impossible! But that was a wake-up moment. A bell clanged, and everything started to shift. I began to notice when critical voices arose and learned how to silence them. I practiced being in the present moment, which led to finding more awareness and peace in my life and more compassion for myself and others. The spiral continues.

What was I reading then? Only one book about what to expect physically. Mostly I read or reread books dealing with women's spirit. *Women Who Run with the Wolves* by Clarisa Pinkola Estes, *Goddesses in Everywoman* by Jean Shinodu, *Anatomy of the Spirit* and *Sacred Contracts* by Carolyn Myss, *The Artist's Way* by Julia Cameron, *Out of the Garden: Women Writers on the Bible*. Several books by Starhawk. Many Buddhist texts, including ThichNhatHanh's *Anger*, Jon Kabat-Zinn's *Wherever You Go, There You Are,* Eckhart Tolle's *The Power of Now*, Matthieu Ricard's *Happiness*. I read a lot of poetry, especially poems by Rumi, Rilke, and Mary Oliver, who asks in her poem "The Summer Day," *Tell me, what is it you plan to do / with your one wild and precious life?*

And I wrote—poems, plays, dreams, journal entries. I dreamed often. All of this led to more discovery. As Frost said, "the initial delight is in the surprise of remembering something I didn't know I knew. ... Writing a poem is discovery."

Experience. Read. Insight. Write. Talk. All part of the spiral of knowing, not-knowing.

I'll end by sharing a few journal entries that capture the sense of yearning, questioning, and claiming I was experiencing during that year of menopause.

5/21/02. When I get an insight while writing—it's so exciting—I write fast before it escapes, then want to share it and hope the other person gets excited by it and then you discuss it, go deeper. ... Next year I might apply for a writer's retreat, go away for a week or two. How I've longed to do that. I feel guilty though. Why do I censor myself? How to break out of being the good girl/mom/wife/worker. I'd like myself more if I could break out of that—I'd be more interesting.

5/24. Dreamt this morning that an owl landed on a tree in our back yard in the daytime. I was in awe of it. It was huge and beautiful and it came so close to me and I wasn't afraid. Owl = wisdom? *Animal Wisdom* says owl is a symbol of the feminine, the moon, and the night. Bird of magic, the darkness within, prophecy.

5/29. I lost my voice by the sea.
By the sea I lost my voice.
The sea keeps doing what it always does. *Hush.*

Debra Kaufman

Forty-Six

I will be turning fifty-five in August and since December 2013, have now gone a full year without my period. Hurray!!! Am single, never had children, never really felt the need, so the whole "I'm no longer a woman" feeling has never been felt by me. I feel free!

Oh, and everyone gets so worked up worrying about the symptoms (hot flashes, irritability, insomnia, etc), but fail to realize that (I believe) only 50% of women even experience ANY menopausal symptoms and of that 50%, many are minor. Myself, my face would flush every once in a while (maybe once every couple of months) and was hot to the touch and would last a half hour to an hour.

While uncomfortable, it really was no big deal. I'm certainly not diminishing others symptoms as I know a few friends that between hot flashes and insomnia, felt pretty miserable.

I'm just saying it may not ever happen to you so why worry beforehand!

Christine M. Kaess

Forty-Seven

As I was a very late in life child with my siblings being old enough to be my mother, not a lot of information was passed down to me by anyone, I'm sad to say. When it came to periods, Mom told me in a way that scared the shit out of me! She said once you start you'll be having periods for around thirty years.

To a child of ten that was like saying – for the rest of my life until I die. And as for menopause? Never, ever came up. I barely recall when she announced at home that this was the last box of Kotex she'd ever need and I just shrugged my shoulders like – whatever.

When my time came around for the passing into another phase of life I didn't have Mom to ask because she had Alzheimer's by this time. So when I asked my sisters they didn't really give me any assistance other than you just make do with it!

I had no one to help me and no one to compare it to. All I had was what I researched on the Internet and a few words from my doctors. It didn't tell me that I would feel squirrely around the edges and to what degree I'd have hot flashes (I had them but not terribly bad, just enough to make sleeping some nights clammy).

I cheated a bit as I said, "Screw this! Give me drugs!" and I was on ERT (estrogen therapy) for a while as my shift in gears came a bit early due to some surgery. I stayed happily on that for some years until the news starting blowing up about the dangers of hormone therapy.

I eventually weaned myself and dealt with getting used to being the new me that I was. The hot flashes weren't fun at all but they weren't debilitating and I had the wisdom enough to wean myself right before winter. Some friends and I used to crack jokes about having power surges and personal heat waves. A good friend used to carry a hand fan with her for a long time. One thing I did notice is that once I was off the hormones my weight did go up and it's been rough trying to drop the pounds.

The bottom line is that everyone is different in how they shift gears with some having a horrific time while others barely register a blip on the radar. My advice is to have a good talk with a doctor you are confident in, read up on the subject a little (though you can overkill on that too), and have a system of support be it a sibling, friends or a mom if you are blessed to have one that talks to you.

Teri Ridley

Forty-Eight

Menopause. I have written and rewritten my piece several times. My goal being to make it light and humorous, but those words just never came. At least not in the way I had envisioned.

Eventually I realized that for me, menopause isn't necessarily light or humorous. It hasn't been the experience I thought it would be and there are many parts that haven't created a lot of enjoyment in this time of my life.

Never did I look at menopause as a new stage of life. It wasn't spoken of in my growing up years. Not by my mother, her mother or my father's mother. For a matter-of-fact, I don't even think I knew it was called menopause until I was well into my teens. It was only referred to as 'the change of life.' How bad could the 'change of life' possibly be? No more periods! That in and of itself should be wonderful, right? Yet this is what I have discovered about the 'change of life' also known as menopause.

Once my younger and more energetic body would bound out of bed ready to tackle the day. Now it drags. One foot slowly creeping out from underneath the covers. The other foot eventually finding its way out of hiding and onto the floor. Shuffling, I walk a few steps into the bathroom in an effort to begin the day.

Previously my nights were full of sleep, but now they are

interrupted by hot flashes and bathroom breaks. Sex, almost non-existent due to the Mohave Desert that has taken up residence in my vagina. And the weight gain. Oh the weight gain!!! It's a vicious cycle, like a roller coaster ride I cannot seem to exit. Not the life I had envisioned.

As the sleepless nights, tired days, and hot flashes wreak havoc on my body, my menopausal mind is being recreated. My mind reflects. I don't reflect on my life as it used to be nor do I consider this to be the end of my life. Instead I simply look at things differently and I find a new perspective. I dream and make plans for things I never would have considered in my younger years. My life, feeling more solid than ever before. A new energy found.

Unique energy! It's different. Not at all like the energy I had in my twenties, thirties or even my forties. This energy comes from deep within me. I pull it up from the depths of my soul. It's what encourages me to rise in the mornings so I can tackle the day. It's what gives me focus and determination.

Somehow, menopause has and is changing me in both good and bad ways. My body, attacking me in cruel ways while my spirit finds peace and contentment in the road ahead.

Each day, a new experience, all because of this change, the change of life.

From Central Illinois, USA,

Debbie

Forty-Nine

When it came to my mid-forties, I was so looking forward to a lightening and eventual cessation of my monthly period. I had been told that since I started relatively late, I should stop relatively early. Sounded good to me!

However, as I progressed through my forty-fifth year, things were not going as planned. Not only was my period heavier, but it was lasting much longer. I was looking for the complaint department!

Finally, when I could take it no longer, I made an appointment with my doctor. After a few tests, my doctor found that my thyroid, which had all but given out on me during the stressful time of my divorce years earlier, was once again acting up.

But how wonderful it was when I started the increased dose of thyroid hormone! Not only did I have more energy, but my period righted itself for about two months, and about the time of my forty-sixth birthday, disappeared completely, never to return! I wish I had known to watch for thyroid problems. I think it's worth keeping in mind.

Bev DiBell

Fifty

Dear Mia and Ava,

As you become Woman your body will go through many changes. You will not only change on the outside but your body within will change as well. Should you want to become Mothers it is something you will be excited for. Choose your mate well. I mean, really think about them as someone you will want to grow old with. You see, after your child bearing years are past, your body will begin to change again. That period, that drove you crazy, will begin to come at times and then other times you will not get it at all. You will have bouts of heavy bleeding as your insides begin to change, see you will no longer have eggs. Be careful as pre -menopause arrives, as you can get pregnant even if your period is no longer regular. Many a baby has been produced during this time. A Change Of Life Child is what I was told they were, by your Grandmother.

I am telling you girls this now because the more you know and the younger you are in knowing the truth of your body, the better you will care for it, or that is my hope.

I asked Grandma a long time ago about the CHANGE and her words to me were "I went through it like a breeze!" As I remember it I saw some tears and a little anger, really just mood swings as your hormones take over and for me one day I had my period and then it was GONE! I loved it! I have no pain and though I have slowed down it has been from injuries and not menopause, you see that is why this book is being written, for us to all share our stories about growing old and the changes our body went through. It seems it has always been a taboo subject never to be spoken of. Most see it as the end of womanhood but for me, your Auntie, it is freedom. Yes the body is changing but I am OK with that. I cannot stay young forever nor do I have the desire to be. I love this part of my life and I want you two to remember forever and ever to enjoy all the stages of your life.

I want you to embrace change. I do not want you to be scared of growing old, as it is a time for you to look back upon all you did and shared with all of those you loved. We are Woman and we are strong. We can have babies or not. We can drive big old trucks or become teachers and share what we know with so many. I want you two to love with all your hearts, yes it will hurt, sometimes more than you think you can stand but you will survive I promise you. Menopause is not scary at all, based on what your grandmother and I have experienced, just the next step in life to pass through.

So live and love and don't use the words The Curse or The Change. Embrace everything that makes you who you are, and know each and every one of us made it through.

We are all writing a little something for those who need to know what it is all about. Some will have stories and poems that will worry you but know yourself and your strengths, for we truly are NOT the weaker sex.

I love you so much and cannot wait for you two to become Woman and pass on what you know about life. This is truly a sisterhood and should never carry shame.

Remember to be kind to yourselves, Mia and Ava.

I have no sister like you have in each other, so I wrote my letter for you.

Auntie Eunice

Fifty-One

I dealt with menopause by eating soya, I grew sage for tea, took black cohash, and supplemented it with high dose capsules.

I used ice cubes on pulse points to cool flushes, dressed in layers that were easily and quickly removable, had a paper folding fan by the bed which had wooden ribs made from sandalwood, avoided spicy food, never had hot drinks in the summer, kept well hydrated, reduced my sugar intake…and a few other things.

But the menopause doesn't stop when your flushes stop. The next thing is bladder control, thinning tissues that cause urinary tract infections, thinning hair, brittle nails, aching joints … I use dandelion and cranberry extract for bladder issues.

Misky

Fifty-Two

The worst part of menopause is that my hips have filled in, and the fat tire around my middle. As if, since I don't have working ovaries, I don't need a hip to balance a baby.

Then came grandchildren who kept sliding down my leg without a ledge to rest on.

MarmePurl

Fifty-Three

Ah, what a time. I'm fifty-six years old, and I started when I was about forty-eight. My monthlies were always quite heavy, but for a few years they were awful and really affected my life. I had to take iron tablets and could never wear white (though I don't mean to be crude). I didn't have any help, just told I had fibroids and to wait till the end of the menopause when they would shrink.

I had really hot flushes. Oh. I remember being out at lovely restaurants and my big red perspiring face looking back at me from some artfully placed mirror, sweat dripping off me. Sleepless nights, first the duvet is on then it's off! But to tell the truth I didn't get mood swings, well, not that I can remember.

I wouldn't have a monthly for about six months then it would come back and stay for about a month, if not longer, then nothing again for about a year then back again. But I have been free now of all symptoms and no monthlies for about four years, I have the very occasional hot flush but nothing like they used to be, so there is light at the end of the tunnel. I didn't take HRT or any meds.

Janet Knight

Fifty-Four

It started early for me – mid forties –
so produced a few frights for a while –
The only problem, the heat:
hot, hot, hot, at the most inconvenient time.

I'd strip down to my bra in the office,
with my assistant on the alert
for visitors, in the outer room.
Her loudly cleared throat was the signal
to throw on my blouse in a rush.

Then I was wed for the second time –
on our honeymoon, wouldn't you know
the last gasp of the curse made a show.

I wanted to please my new husband,
gave up smoking,
took up eating sweeties instead;
put on the pounds with a vengeance,
I must have been weak in the head.

My first-born was planning his wedding
as groom's mother there was action to take:
to reduce from size 16 to 12,
so no more cheese, milk or yogurt —
my near-fatal mistake.

The result of reduction of calcium
makes an awful warning for you.
Don't worry about a bit of fat.
By the time I turned sixty my bones were so thin
that they broke at the drop of a hat.

Starting when you are very young,
eat lots of calcium-rich food,
take weight-bearing exercise all of your life,
to make sure that your bones stay strong.

But all of that is the serious side -
the rest is nothing but positive:
you can have fun
for the rest of your life,
with no tampons and mess
no mood swings,
no period pains,
and, for me, goodbye to migraines,
what's not to like?

ViV Blake

Fifty-Five

What the hell?

My flirtation with pre-menopausal symptoms was self-induced. Or at least coincided with myself ceasing to take birth control pills. My mother was diagnosed two years ago with breast cancer, estrogen-induced. Therefore, I decided I would eliminate the pills I was taking to regulate the estrogen levels in my own body.

I became my very own space heater.

It was July. July in Illinois is H-O-T. I am prone to sweating (versus perspiring), turning beet red and cussing. Suddenly, even in comfortable, air-conditioned settings, I would feel a flush swoosh up from chest to my forehead. In a non-demure manner, I would begin to fan myself, lift my hair off my neck, and look about for the person that must be holding a blow torch nearby. I remember one time, while enjoying a margarita with my sister at our local Mexican restaurant, blurting out, *Holy hell, is it hot in here?*

These flashes interfered with my quality of sleep. I would wake up, throw the covers off, cool down, doze off, then wake up shivering as my body went back to its normal temperature. However, I did not and still do not, want to resume taking man-made hormones. So, I accepted it as a joy of getting older.

Eventually, my body adjusted to being off the pill and life returned to 'normal.' I have just started feeling some mini-flashes resuming. They are not nearly as intense. I believe I may be starting the pre-menopausal stage. We shall see.

For now I am hot & flashy (literally) in Illinois!

Marla Eversole

Fifty-Six

I got off easy. Menopause sneaked in along with my brand new husband's cancer and went unnoticed, or at least undiagnosed. In the months that followed, in another city, doing daily battle with a cruel and mighty tumor, I might wake up soaked in sweat now and then, and my period seemed to have gone missing, but I blamed it on stress and wrenching circumstances. When I did give it serious consideration, I recalled my mother's experience: "Sometimes my forearms would sweat." And indeed, for me it never got any worse than the occasional night sweat (which abated after a few months), and a mid-section that didn't curve inward anymore (when in fact it never had).

I believe in karma, the kind that happens pretty much in real time, assigned to particular events. And so I also believe that – genetics aside – my minor scrape with menopause is what I got in exchange for my husband, who didn't make it. As change goes, for me menopause wasn't a big one.

Teresa Elliott

Fifty-Seven

My mother is still alive and she told me nothing about menopause. I went through menopause very early, at age thirty-nine, as a side effect of IVF. I'd remarried at thirty-six and my new husband wanted children so I went along to the doctor to see if everything was still working as it should. I was sent for an x-ray of my Fallopian tubes. I had an allergic reaction and both tubes were stuffed up…along came IVF. The drugs made me sick and fat for three years. There was an ectopic pregnancy that exploded, leaving me quite ill. Then one day my sympathetic doctor announced that I had gone through menopause. That was the end of the baby idea, just as well probably.

I have been having hot flushes, or flashes as they are called in U.S. for more than twenty years. I don't think they will ever go away. I refuse to take HRT as an early bout with that left side effects worse than hot flushes and I don't think we should take it anyway. I can live with hot flushes…if that is the worst life throws at me then that is OK. Menopause is nothing to be frightened of – it is part of life.

I love my life at sixty-one. I miss certain things, but I can do things now that I didn't have time for before. I'm glad I didn't have that child. I have a lovely boy of forty-one, plenty for me. Now I travel, build a garden and have a great time.

Debra Kalka

Fifty-Eight

I was thirty-eight years old when I had my first and only child. Pregnancy was a wonderful thing, especially since it negated the throes of peri-menopause I had begun during the previous year. But pregnancy and then nursing for fourteen months only delayed the inevitable.

I think back now and realize it was not so horrible. But the sleeplessness and heavy, erratic periods seemed horrific at the time I was experiencing the symptoms. Around age forty-five I seemed to hit the peak of the experience. Having a young child was challenging enough! God, having a sense of humor, kept on challenging my endurance. Naps were my salvation. Coffee with mainly female friends became a daily balm. Though on many days, caffeine seemed to enhance the symptoms. Wine in the evening would do the same, but then would also calm my frazzled spirit. I had night sweats, but not too badly. I can only remember having to change my nightgown on a few occasions. I do recall wild dreams, but did not write them down. Perhaps I should have!

I did not seek medical relief, though it was offered by my physician. Instead I tried to eat soy in the forms of edamame for snacking and tofu as my main protein at least twice weekly. I feel that it helped. I focused on healthy routines in meals and exercise. Drinking lots of water, not sodas or sweetened iced tea (I live in the deep South!) helped. Walking daily helped. Sleep – even if only via catnaps – helped. Talking with close friends, our therapy over coffee really helped.

My erratic cycles finally became more regular and much

lighter. I skipped a few cycles in my late forties and then magically they stopped. I was forty-eight. My doctor confirmed my menopause via my blood hormone levels. By this time my daughter had became a teenager, and I was nearly finished with the symptoms. A very good thing, as my daughter would argue over the color of the sky on a blue cloudless day. She still does.

I am fifty-seven now and my daughter will be heading off to college this fall. I am nearly ten years out from symptoms, though I will occasionally have a brief hot flash. Nothing that standing in the freezer at the grocer won't help. (I forgot to mention the daily trips to the grocer's freezer section!) I did crave ice cream & chocolate. I don't think I got over that symptom.

My attitude changed for the better. I learned to say, "No." And not over extend myself, for the most part. Both may be from maturity, but I tend to think they come with the passage through the Pause.

A few years ago, I found that I had a very low vitamin D level and now take a daily dose. My D levels are nearly normal. I wonder now if my menopause symptoms would have been lessened had I begun taking vitamin D earlier.

I guess that covers my ten years. It is not a set point, but a process. I still see lack of sleep as being my worst symptom. I can handle anything if I can get sleep.

GA in GA

Fifty-Nine

To my daughter,

Your grandmother Jennie was born in the U.S. territory of Hawaii to indentured laborers from Okinawa. She was an incredibly self-directed individual who overcame the traumas of being stranded in Tokyo as a teenager during World War II, and being disowned by her parents for insisting that she wanted a college education. She supported herself during her college years and went on to Johns Hopkins to become a registered nurse. Due to a familial predisposition and the traumas of her early years, she struggled fiercely with depression all of her adult life. Your grandmother was of the generation that didn't talk about menstruation and menopause; she preferred to inform her daughters by giving us books and the starter kits that Kimberly-Clark made available. She answered questions only after we made use of the dictionaries and encyclopedias she and grandpa bought for us. While this seems like dodging the necessity of talking about the subject, it saved your aunt and me from misinformation — even if we weren't spared the implied negativity of that approach.

Your grandmother had a difficult menopause and like many women of her generation, had a hysterectomy to bring an end to the heavy, uncomfortable periods and the emotional up and downs that were her experience of menopause in my pre-teen years. She was still estranged from her family at the time and I realize she must have felt alone, and ANGRY. I will never forget the day grandpa came home from work and she told him through clenched teeth, "Today, I had the urge to kill!" Those sharp-toothed words were both the depression and menopause speaking. It took me many years to understand that words like those weren't really always about your aunt or me, and not a result of menopause either.

My own experience of menopause was different. I was perimenopausal in my mid-thirties, five years after your brother was born. Can you imagine starting to have hot flashes so soon? My doctor prescribed birth control pills to manage the symptoms, but by the time I was 38 years old, I was well into menopause. I stopped the birth control pills and chose not to try hormone replacement therapy because of a family history of blood clots. For me, menopause was unpredictable periods, night time hot flashes, insomnia and feeling grouchy because I wasn't sleeping well. The shelves at the drugstores were filled with supplements that claimed to relieve menopause symptoms and I tried many of them. I mourned the loss of my fertility, but was not sad at all about the end to my periods – the last one was over ten years ago! I had an easier time of menopause than your grandmother.

Menopause was the time I redefined myself and what being a woman meant to me.

It was surprisingly hard – and at times I marveled at my superficiality! Youthful beauty no longer has a place in my definition of myself, and I am a lot more comfortable in my own skin these days.

I hope I am still on this earth when you come to the change that is menopause. You already know that nothing that can be described in words is forbidden in our conversations. I look forward to walking and talking with you through that experience.

I will always love and support you.

Mona Baker

Sixty

Journal entries during this time in my life

6/23, two dreams:
　　1) I worked in a hospital. It was very busy. I was a department head and was giving orders, getting things done, making important decisions quickly. People were being treated, I was doing good work. But I realized how frenzied it was. I thought, *It can't stay like this, bad decisions will be made.*

　　2) I was walking through the garden with the kids. We were stepping over plants. Darcy said, *There has to be another way.* I said, *Oh, stop and look!* The yard and garden were like an impressionist painting— shimmery colors, beautiful patterns, sun illuminating the scene, a breeze. We watched, breath-taken. I said *— I've never seen it from this perspective before.*

Debra Kaufman

Sixty-One

I'm sixty-one years old and haven't had a period in fifteen years. I vaguely recall my mother complaining about being 'terribly warm' but it certainly wasn't something she'd speak of openly. I recall her taking me to somebody's house where several of her acquaintances also brought their daughters to watch a movie called *YOUR BODY!* It at least explained the physical changes young girls could expect, but it seems Mom must have thought that that was enough, as she never said anything about the movie afterwards.

I was something of a surprise pregnancy. Mom was thirty-eight when I was born, and my sister and brother are eight and nine years older than I. She did mention in passing that she didn't realize she was pregnant for some time as she thought it was The Change and after I was born she never had a period again. My sister simply stopped having periods when she was thirty-seven. She had always been a 28-day-at-noon type. I, on the other hand, went through several months of extremely heavy periods. When I did seek help the doctor's answer was to put me on birth control pills. It wasn't long after that that things started winding down.

Because I was certain from a pretty early age that I didn't intend to bear children, I actually looked forward to menopause. I didn't marry until I was forty-five and was well on the way to being done with everything. I had always had some mood swings and had bouts of mild depression that I just powered my way through, but after menopause they got progressively worse. In the blink of an eye, I would go from feeling perfectly normal to senseless rage over nothing, or being down so far I could barely speak. I tend to be sarcastic so I've always tried to hold my tongue — what you don't say can't come back to bite you in the butt — I truly don't like hurting people's feelings but it also meant I pretty much kept my own council.

With the pause came hot flashes and night sweats and terribly broken sleep, which probably exacerbated the down moods. I do recall waking one night, so drenched with sweat that my silky red nightie made the sheets pink. Only cotton for me now. I seldom see a doctor, but was so desperate for sleep I finally went. I'd tried so many, many herbal and natural supplements for both menopause and insomnia, but nothing helped. His answer was a prescription for diazepam, for anxiety. While it let me sleep it put me in such a deep dark hole I felt as if I lost all my joy. Nothing, not my dear husband, my gardens or my animals could raise my spirits — so I gave that up. After a few more months of no sleep I went back, and this time we tried a mild antidepressant. While it improved the sleep problem a little bit — I actually do dream on occasion now — it truly helped with the vile moods and most importantly, I got my joy back.

My 'thermostat' is still kind of out of whack. I still get a couple of mild power surges a day, and am usually awakened somewhere around 3am feeling like I'm cooking — but things have calmed down quite a bit. Oddly enough, the symptoms ebb and flow and seem to be cyclical, much like the periods were. I have just resigned myself to spending a lot of time in the wee hours wide awake and being in a perpetual state of Tired. I had always been quite thin but now have acquired a 'muffin top' that just will not be pared down no matter how many miles I walk or ride a horse or how many farm chores I do. I have absolutely no libido anymore and intercourse is downright painful, while I feel sorry for my husband I am usually just too tired to care. I am so very lucky that he is so very understanding. Perhaps it is because he's ten years older than me, and watched his first wife suffer with ovarian cancer for six years before succumbing at forty-nine or that we have supported his second daughter through three bouts with that same monster. (She's doing well- knock on wood.)

Whatever makes him what he is we are both retired and enjoying life. We both might have the aches and pains that come with 'the golden years' and I might always suffer the after effects of menopause but life is good, you just can't sweat the small stuff.

Cheerio

Sixty-Two

Methinks I have always believed in the importance of mind-body medicine but no more so than in the hormonal world of puberty, childbearing and menopause. I honestly think we pass these natural milestones in life according to how our life is enveloping us just at that moment. Perhaps my happenings versus my mother's are a good example.

Mother's change of life began within a year of her oh-so-unhappy arrival in Australia after the end of WWII. I was far too young and immature to realize what she was going through. Before losing her home country and her way of life to become a political refugee because of Communist terrorism, I guess she had led the charmed life as the wife of a very up-and-coming army-law personality with a beautiful home, abundant staff and a cafe society persona. Suddenly she had to try and survive in a single room with the contents of a single suitcase and no social position at all, without understanding English nor how any of her neighbours lived.

She spoke four other languages and had worked as a brilliant financial controller in her youth – but English was not on the syllabus in NE Europe of the time. Dad worked at a necessary factory job for unholy hours. I was doing well in a totally alien but fascinating world at school. She struggled alone at home.

The local shopkeepers thought she was a joke in her high heels, formal dress, hat and gloves and oft I had to be the one to have to do the shopping after school with her in tears. She could not believe so many foodstuffs taken for granted back home were not known or available here.

Australia seemed to be the most horrid and primitive backwater in the world.

I remember accompanying her to the only Estonian physician allowed to practice here some fifty kilometres away from home. Having a highly elevated blood pressure, she was put onto a wicked cocktail of vicious tablets to cope with that and the menopause, which had struck her.

I had just entered puberty myself with no major hassles bar suprapubic pain for the first day or two that one time a month. Hate to think I was far from kind when she would stop every five minutes or so on the street to wipe her face, steady her step and whisper "I just cannot take any more." I DO remember saying, and more than once, "Mom, everyone is looking, you are embarrassing us." Puce in face, covered in sweat and probably dizzy to boot, this new alien land surely must have seemed horrendously unkind to her! I do not think she suffered from mood swings . . . life had just become an intolerable depressive pain, which seemed to last for years.

By the time I was about forty-nine I was not surprised when symptoms suggesting change of life began to appear. We were a very social 'lot' on The Shores and the first few times one of my dinner party partners quietly handed me a big handkerchief winking and saying "Hot here tonight!" I knew I too was turning noticeably puce!! Must have been the wine or the grins or whatever – offended I was not . . . touched when quite a few quietly asked: "Are you managing?"

Of course I was . . . but knew of friends who did have problems. Luckily I had never had an iota of PMT before and my temperament stayed on an even keel all along .

And then a miracle of life appeared – one early New Year I was part of an Estonian Summer University Seminar down south . . . well, he got out of his car, all 6 feet 5 inches of him . . . and though there were over two decades twixt us 'the wrong way about' he was to turn into the love of my lifetime!! For over four years of my menopause!!! Who on earth had time to worry over hot flushes or even horrendous bleeds every few months. I had a delightful local friend/GP who would insist "Eha, time for TLC at the Mullumbimby Hospital, have a D&C, and let the kitchen staff pamper you for a few days."

I 'knew' I was not 'old,' I 'knew' I was 'attractive,' I had a wow of a time even if the future logically looked bleak! Thank you Higher Powers, wherever and whatever you are. Well, when we were certain the menses had stopped, we all were jubilant. No more fear of pregnancy . . . we knew the relationship could be but temporary, I knew I had huge financial challenges ahead, but unlike for my mother, for me these were to be the most fascinating years of my life.

Difficult days were ahead, difficult years of changes and moves until I decided to regroup here in the country where these changes seem to have become permanent. A decade plus ago I was told I had ovarian cancer: a mistake doctors made viewing a huge cyst I had developed. After that they missed a double breast cancer . . . somehow one managed the mastectomy too. And have so far lived to tell the tale.

Menopause for me was to be the least problematic change of my lifetime.

Eha Carr

Sixty-Three

My story is very short – having gone through menopause in my mid-fifties with very little bother. I used to get headaches two to three days before a period came and then I got headaches when the period would have started but it didn't. This went on for about eighteen months until I realised that I was not menstruating any more. Yay!!

No hot flushes or such discomforts, although I am told I got rather moody from time to time. "Who, me?" I started having periods when I was about eleven years old, and a year later they stopped for about a year. My grandmother, who used to look after me, died – and I think the emotions around that caused my periods to stop.

She never told me anything about what to expect, just presented me with a pack of pads when I first saw blood. Oh, how good it would have been to have had the Internet then and be able to find out what was happening. Being an only child, and there just being me and my Dad, with no other immediate family, it was rather scary at times. People did not discuss such things in the 50's in the UK. However, I did have a lovely lady doctor who gladly showed me how to insert a tampon. Such freedom after those horrible pads.

That is really all my story surrounding menopause, so whilst it isn't amusing or confronting in any way, I hope it helps.

Joy

Sixty-Four

If I had a sister…

If I had a sister she would understand why I have to embrace suffering all the menopausal symptoms.

A little over three years ago, I was diagnosed with breast cancer – many of the symptoms were being put down as probably menopausal – despite having regular periods. The breast cancer was treated, and then my body decided to have another go at trying to end my time on this earth – an overactive thyroid the cause. The thyroid problem was also put down to menopausal symptoms, fortunately a doctor decided to test for an overactive thyroid, which probably saved my life, and now I am actually in The Change.

My symptoms have so far been pretty mild compared to many of my friends, I am sure there is worse to come but when I feel down or fed up, I just remember I am here to feel the hot flushes/flashes, night sweats, headaches, heavy periods, mood swings and for me the worst thing- the weight gain.

I am now trying to work out if I should have HRT, which has made it so much easier to bear for lots of women as there are two schools of thought on this for breast cancer survivors.

Fortunately I have the support of a wonderfully understanding husband (and he really does need to be) and two wonderful daughters. My mother is very open and often very blunt when talking about her experience of the menopause, which is great, hopefully I will be the same with my daughters when they need me to be.

So my advice to a sister would be double check it is the menopause and if it is seek medical advice and help if you feel you need it and be thankful that have reached this time of your life as so many have not.

Alison B

Sixty-Five

What does it mean that in my dreams I am always getting ready to move?

I have lived in a total of seven houses if you don't count short-term rentals, and I don't. Five have been as an adult, two as a child. When I was three my parents moved from a home they loved into one that was nothing special, but in a better school district. My mother lived in that house, the one she never grew to love, until the day she died.

Seven houses is surely enough, for now anyway. And yet at night I wander through house after house trying to find whatever it is my sleeping self is looking for. Usually the homes don't feel familiar, but sometimes they do. Every once in a great while I find myself back in the house where I grew up, and I sit on that plaid Herculon sofa and talk with my parents, both gone for so long now. I always wake from those dreams with a smile.

When I try to think back on what my mother told me about *going through the change*, as she called it, I remember only jokes about hot flashes, and good natured complaints about the hormones they gave her to help with the hot flashes. I think I imagined *going through the change* as something you went through and emerged from unaltered. Like going through a tollbooth or a tunnel or a rainstorm. Menopause was a *pause*, a short-term rental, not a new address. And I honestly can't recall my mother doing anything to dispel that image. She aged as she lived, with a wry smile on her face, waving around a cigarette, laughing at most things, shrugging off the rest. She had her heartaches, some secret, some painfully public, but I don't remember ever seeing her cry.

I was twenty-six when my mother was fifty-one, the age I am now. When I look back at old photos, I think I look younger at fifty-one than she did, but I would think that, wouldn't I? None of us is ready to watch ourselves grow old. Now that I'm the one *going through the change*, I wish I'd paid more attention to my mother's experience, but there are lots of things I wish I'd done differently. Wishes and regrets are a part of life, and that one, although on the list, isn't one that keeps me awake at night. Besides, is knowing what lies ahead really that important when you're approaching the unavoidable?

My house is quiet now, my children grown and gone, and my time divided easily between work and play and rest. It would be nice to have my mother around now that I have the time and the quiet to listen more carefully to her stories. But she died when I was thirty-three, my youngest child only two.

It was years before I stopped picking up the phone to call my mother to tell her about something funny that had happened. If she were still here I'm sure I'd call and complain about my hot flashes and she'd tell me to run cool water on my wrists or eat soy or whatever advice a mother should give a daughter. And I'd tell her about my dreams, about how even though I'm happy enough where I am right now, I can't seem to stop house-hunting in my sleep. I'm betting she'd understand. She'd wave that cigarette around and laugh and laugh. I'd like to think so, anyway.

Melissa DeCarlo

Sixty-Six

In the humid human jungle, there is a rapacious beast that cheerily attacks and devours the happiness of many a poor body.

Menopause. Yessiree, I'm sufficiently past the mid-century mark to be personally acquainted with the joys of middle – and slightly past middle – age. I managed, thanks to magical genes, good luck, or some jolly combination of the two, to enter into the mysterious temple of Menopause well ahead of the dull-normal average age of fifty-one. I guess my body just couldn't wait for the fun. Forty years old? Yay! *Sure*, I can go right ahead and get on that crazy train.

My doctor thought I might just be a fanciful young'un, imagining I was wandering into menopausal territory at the tender age of forty. Until I described my hot flashes. She already knew about my newly accomplished slide to the bottom of a depressive slope, a thing that (while it is seldom developed in complete isolation from other qualities or characteristics of health issues) can sometimes also be a symptom of menopause. She was *not* one of those dismissive, demeaning doctors who would've opted to imply that I was some kind of hysteric or stupid person. So she did a little checking into my state of being in other ways and lo, what I was experiencing was indeed early onset menopause. Or perimenopause, to be more medically precise.

Anyway, I'm now well past a dozen years of this fun and am still here to tell the tale. What's particularly interesting to me is that it's not wildly improbable that I'm, well, okay. I think I might've bought, at least a little, into the popular mythology that makes menopause universally into a horror of monstrous proportions. I will never minimize the true suffering that some women experience during menopause, a very real horror. But me, I've spent over a decade in the strange land of menopause, and I'm still ticking along.

One thing that I have working in my favor, besides that I have relatively few symptoms and lots of blessed good luck, is that I have great support. I have always existed in the midst of a family, friends and acquaintances where topics of real and everyday importance are generally discussed in real and everyday ways. No big deal. Imperfections, illness, death, human failings, and yeah, menopause. These are all realities and unavoidable. Sometimes painful, sometimes inexpressibly difficult, ugly, terrifying, awful. But in all of that- normal. So why would we be so foolish as to pretend otherwise, to let them loom, magnified, as the sort of thing we can never name, let alone discuss, with others who are statistically likely to have shared the experience and might even have wisdom to share in how to survive?

I'm trying to be smart about protecting myself from the bone density loss that is typical of many women in menopause, taking supplements and keeping active as my doctors have recommended. As an exercise hater, this one isn't easy for me. I do keep current with monitoring and treating my depression so that I am sad only, what seems to me, to be a pretty normal amount and about pretty average things. Not depressed in extreme and unhealthy and perniciously persistent ways as I was before I began finding the right health regimen of counseling and medication to keep me on a better path. I use extra skin moisturizer and the occasional application of hair cream rinse because despite having been an almost magically oily youth (and having had to battle high-grade acne as a result) I do find that in my advancing years I now have fairly dry skin and hair.

The big annoyance that remains for me is that my internal thermostat broke when I turned forty. My body forgot how to regulate its own temperature, so now I can go in a matter of seconds from the freezing Undead-body temperature I was so long accustomed to experiencing in pre-menopausal years, to the miracle of my torso becoming a microwave oven and then right back again in a few minutes. Sometimes many times a day. This fun, for thirteen years and counting. And yet I am not a wreck.

The best defense I've found thus far is a simple little device that is a hybrid of that grand old invention, the hot water bottle, and the slightly newer iteration of the athlete's curative bag of ice, a flat water-filled-sponge-containing rectangular envelope thingy that goes by the euphonious rapper-appropriate name of *Chillow* (trademark registered) and can be laid across my overheated midriff when I can't seem to get my inner temperature moderated. It's no cure, but it helps, and help is far better than misery. Even a good old-fashioned accordion-folded fan fluttered southern-belle-style beats undue discomfort.

I would never be so self-indulgent or ridiculous as to call my sufferings massive or anything nearly as important as those of women who endure the real pain possible with menopause and its related conditions. That would be both silly and hypocritical. I'm average, plain, simple, and normal in this experience, even when I'm not exactly on the middle line of the statistical charts. But I can assure you that if you are heading into menopausal territory or someone you know is on her way, there is a path through this particular jungle and you need not be devoured by the beasts met along the way.

See you on the other side of the (very sweaty) swamp.

Kathryn Sparks

Sixty-Seven

All Of A Piece

What a strange word – menopause. The "meno" part, I'm sure, comes from the word menses. It's the second part that baffles me – "pause." There is the implication that the first part is coming back, that this is but a momentary respite from the cramping and the bleeding and the bloating, a temporary break from the inherent bitchiness caused by the cramping and the bleeding and the bloating. That can't possibly be right so from the start, I knew that this whole menopause thing was going to be a "figure it out as you go" kind of a deal. I was actually okay with that. It's how everything of a "female" nature has always been for me.

I grew up in an era where such things were rarely talked about, and then only in veiled references that I was neither old enough, nor clever enough, to figure out. Periods were my mother's "time of the month" or my grandmother's "lady time." There were no mother-daughter talks, no explanations. It was all very mysterious. I'm not criticizing mind you; it was a time when manners ruled and polite conversations did not include body parts. On those rare occasions when you really needed to ask about them, they were spoken of in hushed tones, as if we were the keepers of ancient secrets.

And so began my journey of female uncertainty. Puberty quickly and unexpectedly turned me from adorable to

awkward. I lived through the onset of periods I didn't know were coming, which, by the way, arrived on the same day as my very first summer pool party. I also managed to survive that little humiliation as well.
I learned what sex was from my very best friend at the park one afternoon and was so completely grossed out that I threatened to never speak to her again if she didn't take it back. Of course, I found out years later that I was completely wrong about that one. (Note to self – apologize to very best friend.)

I grew into a young woman, married, became pregnant. And I still had no clear idea of what I was doing. Case in point – the ridiculous notion that no matter how much weight I gained, it would magically go away when the baby came. That one was particularly disappointing.

As the years passed, I became comfortable in the not knowing. I had learned to trust my instincts, to not worry so much about what I didn't know. And I was beginning to suspect that whether I figured things out or not, my body knew exactly what it was doing.

It was right about here that I began to hear murmurings about my mother "changing." A fairly frightening thought given the fact that I liked her just the way she was. It was whispered, of course, and I didn't dare ask her but looking back, I remember being concerned by some of her behaviors. She'd gotten a little moodier, a little quicker to cry. I didn't like it but I honestly didn't have a clue why it was happening. And she never said a word. Over time, she leveled out, she had not changed enough that I no longer recognized her, and I didn't think about it again. I suppose it must have occurred to me that she was going through menopause but if that were the case, it didn't seem all that big a deal. Besides, it was years and years before I would need to worry about it. I was young and as the young are wont to do, did not give my own aging process a second thought.

But time passes and babies become toddlers and then teenagers. Flawless skin begins to show faint lines and strands of gray seem to appear overnight. Still, this mysterious thing called menopause never occurred to me. I was getting older to be sure, but at the mid-point of my 40's, I certainly wasn't there yet.

Or so I thought.

Let me introduce you to my little friend, "perimenopause." I began to notice a few vague symptoms, all of which were fairly easy to explain away. My reliable periods had become not quite so reliable, I was gaining weight – not a lot but enough that the previously successful "cut back on the eating and exercise more" no longer took care of it. More headaches, other things that ached for no apparent reason, fatigue – a lot of that actually. When it got annoying enough, I went to the doctor and it was then that I learned that I was in this other strange thing called "perimenopause." And yes, I had to look it up. Apparently the prefix "peri" means "around or about or approaching" as in about to pause menses, or, as we say here in the south, fixin' to.

So there I was, fixin' to start menopause. Except I didn't. Not for six more years. Still had all the annoying things I couldn't figure out but that's it. It didn't turn in to anything. It just was. The unpredictable became normal for me, the uncertainty not so bad. Until, after six years of being lulled into some sort of false sense of security that this was as bad as it would get, it got worse. Here and there, a little at a time.

The headaches were more frequent, the weight gain more stubborn, the periods more erratic, but right there, that last one, I should have paid more attention to. They weren't just unpredictable, they were worse, much worse. Discomfort turned to pain, pain to what I can only imagine a stabbing ice-pick might feel like, and not to gross you out worse than my little playground friend, the bleeding turned to something akin to hitting an artery.

We're going to skip over the next part, which involved several ER trips, lots of tests, and many quite lovely drugs, to the day menopause became not just something I was approaching but something that had arrived. I had a hysterectomy and, let me tell you, it's bad enough to start losing estrogen slowly over time. It's something altogether different for you to go to sleep with it, and wake up without it.

My very competent, very compassionate, very male gynecologist tried to warn me, which in retrospect is pretty funny. Still, he all but insisted I start taking hormones immediately. "It's going to get bad," he warned," Really, really bad. Let's just go ahead and prevent that from happening, shall we?"

Well, no we shan't actually. Unlike 50 years ago, when there was no Google available for me to find out why I was bleeding every month, or that sex wasn't gross, or that you can't gain eighty pounds, have a six-pound baby, and not come home with the extra 74, I could find out for myself.

A week of research and a history of breast cancer in my maternal gene pool made the decision a piece of cake. I'll never forget my doctor's reaction when I told him I wouldn't be putting synthetic hormones in my already seriously confused body. "Okay, dear. It's your decision," he said as he patted my hand. "You give me a call when you change your mind."

So here I am, squarely in the middle of full-blown menopause. Yes, weight these days is way easier to gain than lose. I've been told that I can be a smidge moody, although I don't see it. The hot flashes are bad, I'm not gonna lie, and night sweats are completely miserable. There have been more nights than I can count when I wake up soaking wet and start flinging off blankets and sheets and peeling off clothes. Note for future reference – do tell your husband or significant other that when you start peeling your clothes off in the middle of the night in your fifties, it does NOT mean the same thing that it did in your twenties.

But it's not all bad, honestly, it's not. For me, a little St. John's Wort here, a dash of Black Cohosh there, the thermostat set on 50 degrees year round, and it's manageable. The one great big glaring advantage is that there are no more periods. Ever. No more PMS, no more bleeding, no more bloating, no more cramping. There is no more need for birth control, which is a nice benefit once you get over the fact that there are also no more children.

Maybe the best part of it all is that it didn't occur until I reached an age where the vanities of youth were no longer high on my list of what matters, when strands of gray became glistening silver threads and wrinkles around my eyes, lovely reminders of spontaneous joyful laughter. It came when I was finally comfortable in my own crazy unpredictable body.

So yes, while it sometimes seems completely unfair that we have all these confusing, and at times frightening, physical changes throughout our lives, I wouldn't trade places with the opposite sex for anything in the world. It is all of a piece and these miraculous, ever-changing bodies know exactly what they're doing. They shelter and sustain the glorious, mysterious creatures that we are.

I don't know about you, but I rather like being glorious.

Sheryl Rider

cecilia b. w. gunther

Sixty-Eight

menopause is hot
burning from the inside out
flush blush sweat and melt

Beth Kennedy

Cecilia (Part Two)

The day I saw The Menopause begin for our Mum was at Mass one warm autumn day. You will have been too little to remember. I know I had Joe on my hip, though he was big enough to walk. So you cannot have been more than ten. I must have been fourteen.

Mum and Dad loved to take us all to Mass every Sunday. They were so proud of their tribe. There were six of us children. Mum would stride up the aisle in her brown court shoes, her head always high, perfectly turned out of course. She wore greens and browns and linen blues, always understated, and always well fitted. Always sheer pantyhose. She was proud as Punch.

She had started to struggle with weight gain and was living on coleslaw and 'that hippy food' that had become the rage then, plus she chewed on strange little appetite-killing toffees you could buy at the chemist. (They were later banned by the Health Department.) She had taken to keeping a big bottle of children's cough mixture in the door of the pantry for a quick swig straight from the bottle when she started to feel a little overwhelmed. (A treat I have to admit I sneaked for myself every now and then when it was my turn to be a harassed mother.) The cough mixture was stored right next to the appetite reducing toffees with other things that we were Not Allowed To Touch. She was in her early 40's then, her short hair was turning grey, and to her gentle chagrin, it was salt and pepper gray, not a gorgeous pure white like Grandma.

She always set it with her fingers into corrugated waves like a dented helmet. She taught us to smooth our skirts beneath us as we all sat filling one pew in the church.

We would follow her into the beautiful old building that we had known all our lives, then file into one of the long, golden bottom-shined pews. Us three girls would smooth our skirts the way she'd taught us and sit. The three boys just plonked themselves down. Mass was her quiet time. Her second home was that church.

Do you remember it — right next to the square, surrounded by huge old palm trees with spiky trunks you could climb on for a dare? It was a tall wooden building with the highest of old fashioned steeples. It has always interested me how American barns and European churches are so much alike. Both full of air and muted sounds. The vaulted ceiling soared up, sheaves of timber locking and interlocking, weaving up towards the sky of prayer that my mother was building. Cow people milling about below. Murmuring. The old native timbers catching rays of colour and fiery dance from the tall magnificent stained-glass windows. The priest in his robes made from donated wedding dresses. It was more cathedral than church in my memory, though I was young and admittedly not very tall.

We would gaze at the horrific Stations of the Cross lining the walls with more blood and torture than really should have been appropriate for children our age.

On that Sunday after Mass was finished, the congregation began to file out, their heads held at that particular tilt that looks smug but is really just slightly dazed, the women with eyes now calmed. (This was the one hour in the week that they could just sit – and stand and kneel, but you know what I mean.) We watched the people leaving wondering when Mum was going to give us the signal to move. Then I noticed that Dad and Mum had their heads together talking to each other instead of nodding and smiling to their friends. This was unusual. Mum never talked inside the church. Abruptly Dad stood and, leaning past Mum, indicated to us to follow him. Mum remained sitting in her pew, her body awkward. Then Dad caught her eye and raised his chin to the side door. She nodded, her mouth set shut. A firm line. We all filed back out, climbing over Mum who slid her knees sideways very slightly. We shuffled impatiently after the last of the congregation, trying to catch up with Dad, who had you and our little brother alongside him. The others ran ahead. I picked up our smallest brother and perched him on my bony hip. I can still feel his strong little legs wrapped around me. He was likely to get out of control if hurried. Prone to tantrums. So I carried him everywhere much to Mum's despair.

At the main church doors, I could not see past the wall of people's backs. So I stalled, thinking I might turn back and leave with Mum. Even as Joe on my hip continued to drift forwards, my body twisted drifting back. I was slightly unbalanced from his weight, and hefting him again with one arm, my eyes searched back into the church for Mum. The church was empty now. She looked small and forgotten way back in her seat. I looked carefully at her as the swinging doors wheezed shut, closing on the last of the whispering people, and the stillness washed past us like a satin broom. Smoothing the air.

She was still sitting in the pew, facing forward to the altar. She cocked her head. She could not hear very well but her Self was sweeping the church for stragglers. Then she straightened her shoulders and began to rise from the pew, way off at the front of the church, all alone, dwarfed by the massive pillars. She rose gathering her brown leather handbag and gloves, reaching for the pointed end of the pew with her left hand to help herself straighten. She wore a pale faun skirt and that perfect cream silk blouse that I still have in the big trunk, her green cardigan settled just so on her square shoulders. She stepped out into the aisle, genuflected, and as she straightened and turned to walk towards the side door, with her head still held high, I saw that the back of her skirt was deeply stained with wet, red blood. I blinked and shifted Joe onto my other hip, twisting so he would not see. I watched her briskly disappear into the small alcove that preempted the elegant side door. I froze there in the back of the church, Joe jiggling on my hip trying to move me along, he leaned forward to steer me out of the church door with his weight, angling me about like a horse. I whirled, my arm tightening around him, my hand – fingers splayed – shoving the towering wooden doors open, and we hurried to catch up with Dad and our brothers and sisters who were already at the side door with the van.

It was that winter that her glide began to crack and her confidence stumbled. Her temper flew right off the handle and straight at our heads more and more often.

She did not get up in the mornings to see us off to school anymore. I think she bled heavily during this time, spent many of her days in bed or sitting with magazines. Our Middle Sister and I slowly took over the housework, and I think, though I am not sure (how does one forget these things?), that she had a hysterectomy soon after, and the slow descent into cancer began.

The furies. I know you remember those. The night Dad took Mum by the shoulders – she was shaking, gutted with fury – and told her quietly that he thought she should go back to bed, go to the bedroom now. The sea at high tide below the big glass doors, whispering things I could not quite hear, following her bare footsteps down the stairs. Currents running through the room I could not net. You, wide-eyed with fear right up against the wall. Poor Little Sister.

To pull things from our memories like this is fraught with despair and wishes. Do you think that this anger was caused by The Menopause or the creeping cancer? It was not like her. It did not belong with how she saw herself. She was so bright and so loved. I think it was the beginning of The Menopause.

However, hindsight is not necessarily a reliable sight at all.

I always thought it was so sad that she died during what I think was her perimenopausal stage. Well of course it was sad that she died at all, but – as my best friend told me one time – you either get old or you die, but to die when you are enduring the heat of your body burning itself into a new shape without ever having the chance to begin your journey with that new shape seems deeply unfair. The drugs for the cancer would have stopped any natural progression in her body. I am positive that if the cancer had not interfered she would have beaten that bloody path to calm. Right through menopause and out the other side. Different, but painting again and writing more.

So I think that Mum must have begun The Menopause cycle in her early to mid-forties. Mum died so young. She told me to tell everyone she was forty-nine because it sounded so much more tragic, but really, she was fifty. I told her I would say she was forty-nine, but I was a terrible liar. She looked at me from her favourite soft flat pillow, her green eyes with those little gold flecks glistening through the stink of pain, and said, "I know." Then she smiled her little 'trying not to laugh at you' smile.

Right, enough of that, we are talking about menopause not dying mothers. I am off to skim this morning's cream into the butter churn, pick the greens for dinner, weed one more row, mow one more lawn, repair the hole in the chook run, clean Aunty Del's pen, train another row of grapes, milk my bad tempered cow Daisy, feed the fattening pigs and chickens the milk, bring the washing in off the line and throw it on the couch, then get dinner on the table (roasted asparagus, roasted onions with honey, grass fed steak seared in my own butter, rosemary potatoes and as many fresh greens as I can fit on the plates). After we have eaten, I will wash up, dry up, put a load of laundry on and with my glass of wine I shall return and finish this letter to you.

Okay, I am finished. What a deep relief it is to sit down at the end of the day. I get very tired sometimes working out here by myself. However, everything is stowed away, the animals are fed, the husband is home from work and fed and in bed. Back to just me again. Back to us.

Now where were we? Mum and The Menopause, or perimenopause or whatever the word is. In all, I think menopause caused her to have a very bad temper at times, bleed heavily; she was always terribly tired and began to battle weight. This is about all I can find out by sifting through my own colander of a brain. So, since we know so little about Mum's dealings with The Menopause, I shall try to piece together my own experiences for you.

I literally forgot about menopause. I have a terrible memory for stuff like that. Most of the time I cannot even remember my own age! I was feeling dizzy on and off when I was living in London in my forty-something years and just thought vaguely that I was dying of something – you know I never go to doctors. Mum died young, and I just assumed I would too. I ignored it. As you do. The dizziness still comes occasionally, usually when I am climbing up the ladder in the barn with a bucket of water for the peacocks. Most unfortunate.

Sometimes my face will get hot, but usually in margarita season. If I sleep under anything but cotton or wool, I will sweat dreadfully, but I have always been like that. I used up all my rages as a young, single mother with too many children when 'potatoes were my best friend' (we will get to that book another day), so I do not get angry often. There is no one to get cranky with, out here, anyway. My husband is gone 12 hours a day, my children are dotted all over the world, I am a recent immigrant to America, and I have no old friends to have arguments with knowing they will forgive me. So, my moods are fairly calm, though I will sulk. But I don't think we can blame sulking on The Change! I don't think. Do you think?

I do have a memory problem, but I can't blame that on menopause either. I have always been absent-minded. It's not like I forget to milk the cow or anything, but sometimes I forget to eat, and it keeps me thin walking everywhere twice to collect the things I forgot the first time. I make lists then lose the lists. I walk into rooms with no earthly clue why I am there. I have decided the memory-loss thing is so our brains can have a rest. I have a very rest-filled brain.

Years ago when my children were babies, I still went to the Doctor, a dear man he was (when he retired from being a doctor, I retired from doctors). This must be 26 or so years ago now. Anyway, I said to him, "I keep forgetting things." As though this was something he could cure. "Were they important?" he said. He looked at me as I thought about the question. I moved the baby from one knee to another and reached down to pull the toddler from under his desk as the toddler's older brother finally finished dragging a chair to the door handle, opened the door to the corridor, slid down off the chair and slipped out the door, looking for his even older brother who had elected to stay in the play area out in the waiting room.

We both listened to him toddle to reception and engage the Nurse in babble.

"I don't know," I said, reaching down for my bag, baby moving in unison with my body, bowing to the floor then back up. "I can't remember."

"Well then," he answered with clarity. Then he went on to tell me that if I lost any more weight he was going to put me in the hospital. "Who will mind the babies if you do that?" I asked, replacing the chair against the wall. I was a divorced woman after all. "I will." He said. I loved that man.

Anyway, in the last year my period has gone missing for months at a time (I am fairly sure I am fifty-three but you know how I am with numbers). I have no idea when my last period was, about six or seven months ago, I think, though I have never been much good at tracking them. They never got heavy or anything, just stopped. I still pack the Cowboys. (My students used "Cowboys" as a code word for tampons). I sometimes get tingly feet, tickly, jiggly, I cannot-stay-sitting-down feet. And like I said, my face and hands get hot flushes, but it is intermittent. The hot flush in my face seems to be on hiatus, but my hot hands return every now and then. And I cannot stand cats winding themselves about my feet – I hate it now. Too much touching! And of course, the headaches, but I have had them since I was young. I almost always get hot flushes, dizziness, tingly feet and my period when I step onto a plane. Go figure. Menopause in a metal capsule.

So there you have it darling girl. I shall pour myself just one more glass of wine. (I don't have a drinking problem,

I promise!) Then I shall pop this in a big envelope with all the other letters The Fellowship have written for you and send the package off across the sea.

You are important and good. Take care of yourself.

All my love little sister.

Your Big Sister,

Celi